Sports Performance Massage

Sports Performance Massage instructs the student and practising therapist to use a combination of experience and scientific evidence to inform their sports massage practice, particularly when working with athletic populations. Strength and conditioning coaches, managers and athletes frequently ask questions about the best use of sports massage in order to recover more quickly from injury and fatigue and improve performance. *Sports Performance Massage* empowers the therapist and gives them greater confidence by improving their scientific understanding when working with injured or competitive athletes.

This exciting new volume covers all the aspects required to make a highly skilled, confident and employable sports massage therapist. Working with high-level athletes requires an additional skill level compared to working with the general public. Furthermore, advanced massage skills taught in this book, such as soft tissue release and trigger point therapy, are essential when working on muscular adhesions and injured areas. Pregnant athletes, those with disabilities, contraindications and athletes with special requirements have also been considered.

Sports Performance Massage is a learning and research aid for those studying vocational sports massage courses as well as those studying other courses where massage forms part of the undergraduate or postgraduate degree, such as sports therapy, sports rehabilitation, osteopathy and physiotherapy. Unlike other sports massage books, *Sports Performance Massage* has a strong academic focus, allowing the graduate therapist to stay up to date with the latest research in their respective field.

Steve Bedford qualified in Swedish massage in 1995 and in sports massage the following year. Further studies and qualifications have included diplomas in sports therapy and sports injury management; certificates in NLP, clinical hypnosis, cardiac rehabilitation, personal training and mat-based Pilates; and a master's degree in sports performance. Steve has worked at every Wimbledon tennis championships since 1999 and worked two seasons for Arsenal Football Club. He was also the unit lead for sports massage on the University of Bedfordshire's sports therapy undergraduate programme and has been a sports massage tutor at the University of East London and the University of Bath. He has published in peer reviewed academic journals and has completed over 60,000 sports massage treatments during his career.

Sports Performance Massage

Steve Bedford

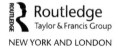
Routledge
Taylor & Francis Group

NEW YORK AND LONDON

First published 2022
by Routledge
605 Third Avenue, New York, NY 10158

and by Routledge
2 Park Square, Milton Park, Abingdon, Oxon, OX14 4RN

Routledge is an imprint of the Taylor & Francis Group, an informa business

Library of Congress Cataloging-in-Publication Data
A catalog record for this title has been requested

ISBN: 978-0-367-61245-0 (hbk)
ISBN: 978-0-367-61239-9 (pbk)
ISBN: 978-1-003-10480-3 (ebk)

DOI: 10.4324/9781003104803

Typeset in Galliard
by Deanta Global Publishing Services, Chennai, India

Visit the Support Material: www.routledge.com/9780367612399

Contents

Figures

Tables

Preface

This book acts as a review and guide for the vocational and university-based student, covering all the competencies required for therapists who have an interest in working with athletic populations. The comprehensive descriptions of commonly used massage techniques and associated modalities inform the reader not only of the science, but also of the techniques' practical application through correct assessment and treatment, with the ultimate goal of keeping the athlete injury- and pain-free and able to perform to the best of their ability.

By reading this book the reader will be made aware of the high demands placed on sports massage therapists working in performance sport by team managers, coaches athletes and other allied sports and exercise medicine professionals. These demands will require you to draw from a wide range of knowledge and experiences. You will need to understand the consequences of overuse (over-training) and the potential risk this brings to the athlete when training or competing, and how massage and other associated modalities may benefit them in order to perform, recover and feel prepared for subsequent performances. To achieve this, you must undertake regular continual training and professional development (CPD) in addition to extensive practice to perfect your sports massage therapy skills. This book offers you the opportunity to enhance both your scientific knowledge and your practical skill base and to apply theory to practice from one of the UK's leading sports massage therapists.

Relevant scientific studies have been identified and examined through the screening of article titles from databases including PubMed, Medline, Sport Discus and Google Scholar. A final reference check using Google Scholar was completed to assess the availability of all articles. Inclusion criteria included research articles in the English language, using only human subjects, where the primary aim of the investigation was to ascertain the effects of massage prior to or following athletic performance, and its physiological and/or psychological effects on performance, recovery and injury. All massage studies included in the writing of this book were inspected to ensure they examined a form of massage consistent with the considered operational definition, where massage is defined as the manual manipulation of the soft tissues, using techniques including either effleurage, petrissage, frictions, myofascial release, soft tissue release, vibrations or tapotement. Other modalities compared to massage in the literature were also investigated, including different forms of cryotherapy, thermotherapy, foam rolling, dry needling, cupping and instrument-assisted massage. In addition, other topics including contraindications to massage, common injuries from a variety of sports, anatomy and physiology are also covered to allow for a greater depth of understanding. The following terms were also investigated and included where appropriate: strength, sprint(ing), flexibility, jump(ing), range of motion (ROM), delayed onset muscle soreness (DOMS), perceived recovery, psychological (perceived) fatigue and performance. For those readers not familiar with research terminology, brief explanations and commonly used abbreviations have been included.

Acknowledgements

This book is dedicated to all the people who have helped me over the years, starting with John Hale. John gave me my first sports massage in the early- to mid-1990s. Whilst waiting for a Taekwondo class to begin, John suggested sports massage could help me with my persistent back pain – he was right! I asked him where he learnt how to massage, and the rest as they say is history. I would like to thank all the therapists and university lecturers I have worked alongside over the years, in particular Chris Salvary – I have learnt something from you all, especially Chris. To Lisa Allen, I would like to thank you for all your help, kindness, patience and support. A special thank you goes to Helen Cawte Photography for her excellent images used in this book. And finally to Spencer and Jude, every day you make me extremely proud – thank you.

Abbreviations and Glossary

A number of abbreviations are used throughout this book, as they are frequently used in research articles and throughout the wider industry. Below is a list of abbreviations and other terms with brief explanations.

Modalities

CCT   cold compression therapy.
CG   compression garment.
CWI   cold water immersion (ice bath, plunge pool).
CWT   contrast water therapy (alternating between hot and cold).
WBC   whole-body cryotherapy (cold chambers).

Exercise-Related

ACT   active recovery.
ATP   adenosine triphosphate. A high energy molecule that provides energy to drive many living cells, e.g. muscle contraction, nerve impulses.
BMI   body mass index. Divide your weight in kilograms (kg) by your height in metres (m) then divide the answer by your height again to get your BMI.
CK   creatine kinase. An enzyme found in muscle and other tissues. When muscle damage occurs, CK is released into the blood, so it is used as a marker to assess muscle damage.
CMJ   countermovement jump. A measure of lower body power, where the jumper starts from an upright standing position, makes a downward movement by flexing at the knees and hips, then immediately extends the knees and hips again to jump vertically up off the ground.
DOMS   delayed onset muscle soreness from unaccustomed or unfamiliar exercise.
EC   excitation-contraction. The release of calcium begins, allowing cross-bridge formation and contraction. This is coupled to excitation: signalling of action potentials from a motor neuron, starting with signalling from the neuromuscular junction and finishing with calcium release for muscle contraction.
EIMD   exercise-induced muscle damage as a result of eccentric or high-volume loading.
IL-6   interleukin-6. Acts as a pro-inflammatory cytokine and anti-inflammatory myokine. Also plays an important role in acquired immune response by stimulation of antibody production.
IVC   inferior vena cava (compression). When lying in the supine position during late pregnancy the vena cava gets compressed by the uterus.

LDH   lactate dehydrogenase. This is an enzyme required during the process of turning sugar into energy for your cells.

MIF   maximum isometric force. Force exerted by a muscle on an object. When muscle tension changes and the muscle length remain the same, it is described as isometric.

MVC   maximum voluntary contraction. Used as a measure of strength. It is a measure of maximal exertional force or as moment around a joint.

PPT   pressure pain threshold. Defined as the minimum force applied which induces pain. Used in evaluating tenderness symptoms.

PR   passive rest.

RM   repetition maximum. The most amount of weight that can be lifted for a specific amount of movements; for example, 5RM is the heaviest amount of weight an individual could lift 5 times without stopping.

TNF-α   tumour necrosis factor-α. A cell-signalling protein which indicates systemic inflammation in the acute phase.

VAS   visual analogue score. A psychometric response scale (usually between 1–10) is used in questionnaires. It is a measurement for subjective characteristics or attitudes that cannot be directly measured.

WU   warm up.

Massage

AKP   anterior knee pain. An umbrella term which is used to describe patella tendinitis, bursitis, cartilage injury, Osgood-Schlatter's disease, Sinding-Larsen-Johansson disease or maltracking of the kneecap within the femoral groove (chondromalacia patella).

DFM   deep friction massage. A specific connective tissue massage applied transversely to the specific tissue involved, used to increase circulation and break down adhesions and scar tissue formation.

ECRB   extensor carpi radialis brevis. Supplied by the radial nerve and has its origin on the lateral epicondyle and inserts into the lateral dorsal surface of the base of the third metacarpal bone, with a few fibres inserting into the medial dorsal surface of the second metacarpal bone.

GH   growth hormone. A small protein that is made by the pituitary gland and secreted into the bloodstream.

ITBS   iliotibial band syndrome (sometimes referred to as iliotibial band friction syndrome). Previously believed to be an overuse injury of the distal iliotibial band rubbing over the fat pad or lateral femoral condyle. Associated with running, cycling and squatting exercises.

LA   lateral epicondylitis (tennis elbow). An overuse injury to the common extensor tendons (especially ECRB).

MRI   magnetic resonance imaging. A type of scan that uses strong magnetic fields and radio waves to produce detailed images of the body.

MTrP   myofascial trigger point. Hyperirritable spots in the fascia surrounding skeletal muscle that feel like palpable nodules in taut bands of muscle fibre.

MTSS   medial tibial stress syndrome (shin splints). An overuse injury or repetitive-stress (traction) injury of the shin area, causing inflammation on the tibial aspect of the lower leg.

NES   neuromuscular electrical stimulation.

STR/ART   soft tissue/active release therapy. Tension is applied to the affected structure as it is moved from a shortened to a lengthened position.

Research

CI	confidence intervals – how well the sample statistic estimates the underlying population. The interval has an associated confidence level which is most commonly set at 95%.
Hypothesis tests	used to test the validity of a claim that is made about a given population. The claim that is being investigated is known as the null hypothesis.
n	the population/sample size used in the study.
p **values**	helps to determine the significance of results. A small p value (for example, $p \leq 0.05$) indicates strong evidence against the null hypothesis, therefore you reject the null hypothesis. Large p values (>0.05) indicate strong evidence against the null hypothesis.
Sensitivity (true positives)	measures the proportion of actual positives that are correctly identified.
Specificity(true negative rate)	measures the proportion of actual negatives that are correctly identified.

1 Introduction to Sports Performance Massage

The Science and Practice of Sports Performance Massage

Prior to working with elite athletes, therapists need to understand the importance of their own health and wellbeing: the correct set-up of equipment for each individual therapist is paramount as working hours can be both long and physically demanding. Working with top amateur and professional teams and individuals requires a high skill set, experience and the ability to work under high pressure, usually as part of a multi-disciplinary team.

Massage therapy has been around for thousands of years and has been described as a way of enhancing biomechanical, physiological, neurological and psychological wellbeing (Weerapong et al., 2005). Its popularity in the western world is due to the work of Per Henrik Ling (1776–1839) who developed the form of massage now known as Swedish massage. Ling developed a style of massage and exercise to help fencers and gymnasts, gaining international recognition in the process. Many of his ideas have formed the foundations of modern sports massage. Tennis players have been receiving sports massage at Grand Slam tennis events since the early 1960s, prior to it turning professional, and at the 1972 Olympic Games, Finnish track and field athlete Lasse Virén credited receiving deep friction massage with winning both the 5,000 and 10,000 meters. In the 1976 film *A Sunday in Hell*, which followed professional cyclists on the French Paris-Roubaix classic, riders regularly received sports massage and understood its importance for their preparation and recovery. Now it would be uncommon for professional sports teams or athletes not to use sports massage as part of their overall physical wellbeing care plan.

What Makes a Good Sports Massage Therapist?

During sports massage courses, student therapists are taught anatomy and physiology, massage techniques, contraindications and cautions to treatment, alignment and posture and a number of special tests to aid in their treatment planning. Once practising massage, to become a competent therapist, confidence, communication skills, limb handling abilities, injury management, stretching techniques, basic first aid and critical thinking all need to be learnt and updated through regular continued professional development. Other key skills include the ability to build a good rapport with athletes and co-workers, as long hours can be spent with the same individuals during training camps, tournaments or competitive seasons.

Does Therapist Experience Make a Difference?

According to a study conducted by Morasaka (2007), it does. Following completion of a 10k running race, 317 individuals completed questionnaires on their level of muscle soreness at

DOI: 10.4324/9781003104803-1

24 and 48 hours post-race. Runners who received a 12–15-minute massage from a student with 950 hours of training (compared to a student completing 700 or 450 hours) reported a greater reduction in soreness symptoms; from the results of this study it therefore appears experience *could* make a difference. In agreement, Donoyama and Shibasaki (2010) recruited healthy 50-year-old females (n = 8) suffering from chronic neck and shoulder stiffness. Each participant received four interventions: three 40-minute massage therapy interventions, one each by a freshman and a sophomore student studying massage therapy, one by their instructor and one resting control. A visual analogue scale was used to measure neck and shoulder stiffness and state anxiety scores. Salivary cortisol concentration levels and secretory immunoglobulin A were also measured pre- and post-interventions. The authors' results indicated that the visual analogue scale of neck and shoulder stiffness after massage by the instructor was significantly lower than after the other interventions, and the score of state anxiety was also lower than after the resting control.

Why Looking After Yourself Is Important

Physically, sports massage is hard work, especially pre-competition massage and working at major events. For the therapist there are high risk factors for the development of overload syndromes, related but not limited to working in a forward flexed body position with an inclined head whilst performing repetitive movements, with the same joints, involving the same muscles (Więcek et al., 2018). In fact, a Canadian study of 502 massage therapists who answered a survey (Albert et al., 2008) about their musculoskeletal injuries reported a high level of pain and discomfort in the wrist and thumb, followed by the low back, neck and shoulders, respectively.

Jang et al. (2006) investigated the prevalence of risk factors in 161 visually impaired practitioners. Results from this study indicated about 71.4% had experienced at least one work-related musculoskeletal disorder in 12 months. Prevalence rates were: finger or thumb, 50.3%; shoulder, 31.7%; wrist, 28.6%; neck, 25.5%; arm or elbow, 23.6%; forearm, 20.5%; and back, 19.3%. Working duration > 20 years had an adjusted odds ratio (OR) for finger or thumb 4.0–4.5 with 95% confidence interval (CI) 1.5–13.8; client contact > 4 h/day had an adjusted OR for finger = 3.2 (95% CI = 1.3–8.1); and ≤ 7 kg pulp-pinch strength had an adjusted OR for upper extremity = 2.9–3.2 (95% CI=1.2–8.3). Adjusted ORs for lower-back symptoms were 3.1 (95% CI=1.3–7.8) and 3.6 (95% CI=1.4–9.6), respectively, for lack of neutral neck posture and inappropriate working-table height. (A confidence interval refers to the probability that a population parameter will fall between two set values for a certain proportion of times). Research has also shown (Więcek et al., 2018) that during selected classical massage techniques, masseurs perform their work at a typical intensity of about 47% $VO_{2\,max}$, which at the same time corresponds to 75% HR_{max} with an average energy expenditure of about 180 kcal when working at a typical intensity for 30 minutes.

Therefore, the papers by Jang et al. (2006), Albert et al. (2008) and Więcek et al. (2018) highlight the need for good posture, correct plinth height, regular rest breaks (when possible) and good use of bodyweight when treating. In addition, care must be taken not to hyperextend the thumb joint or place excessive pressure on an extended wrist – these are all important factors to remember for the longevity of the practising therapist.

Employment, Equipment and Couch Set-Up

Employment

A number of sports massage therapists will be self-employed, working in a health and fitness club on their own or in an allied health professional's clinic. Therapists usually work either on a room rental arrangement, or the business owner takes a percentage of any monies received (typically ranging from 25–60%). Employment options include working with semi-professional or professional athletes or sports teams, or for a governing body such as the English Institute of Sport (EIS) or Association of Tennis Professionals (ATP). Some business owners, teams or governing bodies will require a certain amount of experience, or for the therapist to be qualified to a certain level (for example, Level 4) and to belong to a massage governing body, e.g. the Sports Massage Association, General Council for Soft Tissue Therapies (GCST) or American Massage Therapy Association (AMTA). It is advisable to work at as many sporting events as possible during practitioner training and during the first few years of qualifying, for networking, to build experience and to gain the necessary level of competence. In addition, whether working as a self-employed or employed practitioner, the correct amount of public liability and indemnity insurance needs to be obtained before treating any athletes. Furthermore, prior to working, advice should be sought from a reputable accountant regarding setting up a business as a sole trader or limited company, and your tax liability.

You will need to promote your services via social media sites and networking at conferences and CPD events, alongside the best form of advertising, word of mouth. If you do a good job, work hard, act in a professional manner, have good timekeeping and gain the confidence of your athletes, there is no reason why your career cannot progress in the direction you wish.

Equipment

If you intend on becoming self-employed or wish to work at sporting events, it is advisable to purchase your own massage plinth, towels, oils and lotions, and couch (paper) roll. When working always make sure you have neutral oils and lotions to avoid skin irritations and allergic reactions (see topical lotions, discussed at the beginning of Chapter 5). Talcum powder can also be used if the athlete has a preference or there are concerns about allergies or leaving residue on clothing. In some treatment rooms and when working at sporting events occasionally there are no handwashing facilities, so using anti-bacterial gel or wipes for cleaning hands and treatment surfaces is necessary. Wherever a therapist works, it is imperative there are adequate supplies of PPE (personal protective equipment) available, to prevent the spread of infectious diseases. All treatment rooms should have adequate ventilation, and all surfaces should be thoroughly cleaned between treatments to reduce the risk of infectious diseases such as Covid-19.

Couch Set-Up

When setting up a treatment couch always make sure it is at the correct height. Standing next to the couch with a straight arm and a clenched fist is a general guide. Always make sure your athlete is well covered and kept warm when possible. The use of a folded towel covering the plinth face hole gives greater comfort during the massage. Couch roll can be used to protect towels, and bolsters (or rolled up towels) can be placed under the feet (in prone) to reduce muscular tension in the hamstring and gastrocnemius area. To prevent knee hyperextension towels or bolsters can be placed under the knees. For athletes with low back discomfort, or larger breasts, additional towels can be placed underneath the abdominals to prevent an increase in lumbar lordosis. A common set-up is shown in Figure 1.1.

The Science: What Does Massage Do?

Massage has long been considered an integral part of sport preparation and conditioning. It assists in recovery (Caldwell, 2001; Galloway & Watt, 2004) and could increase range of

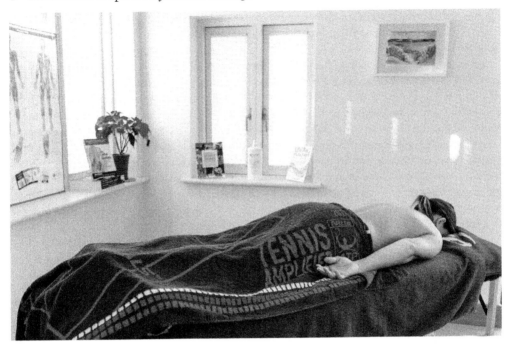

Figure 1.1 A typical portable couch set-up.

motion (Hopper et al., 2005; Arabaci, 2008; Huang et al., 2010; Bedford et al., 2018); reduce the effects of delayed onset muscle soreness (Hilbert et al., 2003; Zainuddin et al., 2005; Mancinelli et al., 2006; Khamwong et al., 2010; Boguszewski et al., 2014; Shin & Sung, 2015; Guo et al., 2017; Holub & Smith, 2017; Dupuy et al., 2018); lower stress and anxiety (Leivadi et al., 1999; Field et al., 2005; Micklewright et al., 2005; Jooste et al., 2013; Zadkhosh et al., 2015); regulate the autonomic nervous system, thereby decreasing levels of cortisol, adrenaline and noradrenaline (Sarli & Sari, 2018); have a positive effect on perceived exertion (Szabo et al., 2008, Bedford et al., 2018); reduce feelings of fatigue (Tanaka et al., 2002; Mori et al., 2004; Ogai et al., 2008; Dupuy et al., 2018; Wiewelhove et al., 2018); promotes faster recovery (Duñabeitia et al., 2019), help with pain and sleep disturbances (Field et al., 2019) and provide psychological regeneration (Hemmings et al., 2000). There is a requirement for greater high-quality research before firm conclusions can be reached on the beneficial physiological and psychological effectiveness of sports massage, both pre- and post-performance, due to conflicting and poorly controlled studies and the lack of decisive evidence.

The Popularity of Massage

Between 1987 and 1998, during 12 national and international events, the total time physiotherapists spent providing sports massage treatment was 24–52.2% (overall median: 45%) (Galloway & Watt, 2004). Now, with greater demand from athletes at major competitions for sports massage, more individual athletes and teams travel with sports massage therapists as part of their sports and exercise medical team; therefore, unsurprisingly, the amount of massage athletes now receive has steadily risen over the last two decades. In a more recent study, Australian team sport athletes utilise massage the most and consider sleep and massage to be the most effective recovery strategies (Crowther et al., 2017). In addition, in a large cohort study (624 patients), 87% of participants with complaints of arm, neck and/or shoulder pain were treated with massage therapy, often in combination with exercise therapy, demonstrating that massage is one of the most popular modalities of choice by therapists and athletes (Karels et al., 2006).

References

Albert, W.J., Currie-Jackson, N. and Duncan, C.A., 2008. A survey of musculoskeletal injuries amongst Canadian massage therapists. *Journal of Bodywork and Movement Therapies*, 12(1), pp. 86–93.

Arabaci, R., 2008. Acute effects of pre-event lower limb massage on explosive and high- speed motor capacities and flexibility. *Journal of Sports Science & Medicine*, 7(4), p. 549.

Bedford S., Robbins D. and Fletcher I., 2018. Effects of an active warm up and warm up massage on agility, perceived exertion and flexibility in tennis players. *Journal of Science and Medicine in Tennis*, 23(2), pp. 16–22.

Boguszewski, D., Szkoda, S., Adamczyk, J.G. and Białoszewski, D., 2014. Sports massage therapy on the reduction of delayed onset muscle soreness of the quadriceps femoris. *Human Movement*, 15(4), pp. 234–237.

Caldwell, E., 2001. *Remedial massage therapy*. Corpus Pub Limited.

Crowther, F., Sealey, R., Crowe, M., Edwards, A. and Halson, S., 2017. Team sport athletes' perceptions and use of recovery strategies: A mixed-methods survey study. *BMC Sports Science, Medicine and Rehabilitation*, 9(1), pp. 1–10.

Donoyama, N. and Shibasaki, M., 2010. Differences in practitioners' proficiency affect the effectiveness of massage therapy on physical and psychological states. *Journal of Bodywork and Movement Therapies*, 14(3), pp. 239–244.

Duñabeitia, I., Arrieta, H., Rodriguez-Larrad, A., Gil, J., Esain, I., Gil, S.M., Irazusta, J. and Bidaurrazaga-Letona, I., 2019. Effects of massage and cold-water immersion after an exhaustive run on running economy and biomechanics: a randomized controlled trial. *Journal of Strength and Conditioning Research*. doi: 10.1519/jsc.0000000000003395.

Dupuy, O., Douzi, W., Theurot, D., Bosquet, L. and Dugué, B., 2018. An evidence-based approach for choosing post-exercise recovery techniques to reduce markers of muscle damage, soreness, fatigue, and inflammation: A systematic review with meta-analysis. *Frontiers in Physiology*, 9, p. 403.

Field, T., Hernandez-Reif, M., Diego, M., Schanberg, S. and Kuhn, C., 2005. Cortisol decreases and serotonin and dopamine increase following massage therapy. *International Journal of Neuroscience*, 115(10), pp. 1397–1413.

Field, T., Sauvageau, N., Gonzalez, G. and Diego, M., 2019. Hip pain is reduced following moderate pressure massage therapy. *Chronic Pain & Management*, 2, p. 17.

Galloway, S.D.R. and Watt, J.M., 2004. Massage provision by physiotherapists at major athletics events between 1987 and 1998. *British Journal of Sports Medicine*, 38(2), pp. 235–237.

Guo, J., Li, L., Gong, Y., Zhu, R., Xu, J., Zou, J. and Chen, X., 2017. Massage alleviates delayed onset muscle soreness after strenuous exercise: A systematic review and meta-analysis. *Frontiers in Physiology*, 8, p. 747.

Hemmings, B., Smith, M., Graydon, J. and Dyson, R., 2000. Effects of massage on physiological restoration, perceived recovery, and repeated sports performance. *British Journal of Sports Medicine*, 34(2), pp. 109–114.

Hilbert, J.E., Sforzo, G.A. and Swensen, T., 2003. The effects of massage on delayed onset muscle soreness. *British Journal of Sports Medicine* 37(1), pp. 72–75.

Holub, C. and Smith, J.D., 2017. Effect of Swedish massage on DOMS after strenuous exercise. *International Journal of Exercise Science*, 10(2), pp. 258–265.

Hopper, D., Deacon, S., Das, S., Jain, A., Riddell, D., Hall, T. and Briffa, K., 2005. Dynamic soft tissue mobilisation increases hamstring flexibility in healthy male subjects. *British Journal of Sports Medicine*, 39(9), pp. 594–598.

Huang, S.Y., Di Santo, M., Wadden, K.P., Cappa, D.F., Alkanani, T. and Behm, D.G., 2010. Short-duration massage at the hamstrings musculotendinous junction induces greater range of motion. *The Journal of Strength & Conditioning Research*, 24(7), pp. 1917–1924.

Jang, Y., Chi, C.F., Tsauo, J.Y. and Wang, J.D., 2006. Prevalence and risk factors of work-related musculoskeletal disorders in massage practitioners. *Journal of Occupational Rehabilitation*, 16(3), pp. 416–429.

Jooste, K., Khumalo, V. and Maritz, J., 2013. Sportmen's experiences at a somatology clinic receiving a sport massage. *Health SA Gesondheid (Online)*, 18(1), pp. 1–9.

Karels, C.H., Polling, W., Bierma-Zeinstra, S.M., Burdorf, A., Verhagen, A.P. and Koes, B.W., 2006. Treatment of arm, neck, and/or shoulder complaints in physical therapy practice. *Spine*, 31(17), pp. E584–E589.

Khamwong, P., Pirunsan, U. and Paungmali, A., 2010. The prophylactic effect of massage on symptoms of muscle damage induced by eccentric exercise of the wrist extensors. *Journal of Sports Science and Technology*, 10(1), p. 245.

Leivadi, S., Hernandez-Reif, M., Field, T., O'Rourke, M., D'Arienzo, S., Lewis, D., Pino, N.D., Schanberg, S. and Kuhn, C., 1999. Massage therapy and relaxation effects on university dance students. *Journal of Dance Medicine & Science*, 3(3), pp. 108–112.

Mancinelli, C.A., Davis, D.S., Aboulhosn, L., Brady, M., Eisenhofer, J. and Foutty, S., 2006. The effects of massage on delayed onset muscle soreness and physical performance in female collegiate athletes. *Physical Therapy in Sport*, 7(1), pp. 5–13.

Micklewright, D., Griffin, M., Gladwell, V. and Beneke, R., 2005. Mood state response to massage and subsequent exercise performance. *The Sport Psychologist*, 19(3), pp. 234–250.

Moraska, A., 2007. Therapist education impacts the massage effect on postrace muscle recovery. *Medicine and Science in Sports and Exercise*, 39(1), pp. 34–37.

Mori, H., Ohsawa, H., Tanaka, T.H., Taniwaki, E., Leisman, G. and Nishijo, K., 2004. Effect of massage on blood flow and muscle fatigue following isometric lumbar exercise. *Medical Science Monitor*, 10(5), pp. CR173–CR178.

Ogai, R., Yamane, M., Matsumoto, T. and Kosaka, M., 2008. Effects of petrissage massage on fatigue and exercise performance following intensive cycle pedalling. *British Journal of Sports Medicine*, 42(10), pp. 834–838.

Sarli, D. and Sari, F.N., 2018. The effect of massage therapy with effleurage techniques as a prevention of baby blues prevention on postpartum mother. *International Journal of Advancement in Life Sciences Research*, 1(3), pp. 15–21.

Shin, M.S. and Sung, Y.H., 2015. Effects of massage on muscular strength and proprioception after exercise-induced muscle damage. *The Journal of Strength & Conditioning Research*, 29(8), pp. 2255–2260.

Szabo, A., Rendi, M., Szabó, T., Velenczei, A. and Kovács, Á., 2008. Psychological effects of massage on running. *Journal of Social, Behavioral, and Health Sciences*, 2(1), p. 1.

Tanaka, T.H., Leisman, G., Mori, H. and Nishijo, K., 2002. The effect of massage on localized lumbar muscle fatigue. *BMC Complementary and Alternative Medicine*, 2(1), p. 9.

Weerapong, P., Hume, P.A. and Kolt, G.S., 2005. The mechanisms of massage and effects on performance, muscle recovery and injury prevention. *Sports Medicine*, 35(3), pp. 235–256.

Więcek, M., Szymura, J., Maciejczyk, M., Szyguła, Z., Cempla, J. and Borkowski, M., 2018. Energy expenditure for massage therapists during performing selected classical massage techniques. *International Journal of Occupational Medicine and Environmental Health*, 31(5), pp. 677–684.

Wiewelhove, T., Schneider, C., Döweling, A., Hanakam, F., Rasche, C., Meyer, T., Kellmann, M., Pfeiffer, M. and Ferrauti, A., 2018. Effects of different recovery strategies following a half-marathon on fatigue markers in recreational runners. *PloS One*, 13(11), p. e0207313.

Zadkhosh, S.M., Ariaee, E., Atri, A., Rashidlamir, A. and Saadatyar, A., 2015. The effect of massage therapy on depression, anxiety and stress in adolescent wrestlers. *International Journal of Sport Studies*, 5(3), pp. 321–327.

Zainuddin, Z., Newton, M., Sacco, P. and Nosaka, K., 2005. Effects of massage on delayed-onset muscle soreness, swelling, and recovery of muscle function. *Journal of Athletic Training*, 40(3), p. 174.

2 Anatomy and Physiology

Muscles

An anterior and posterior view of muscles is shown in Figure 2.1.

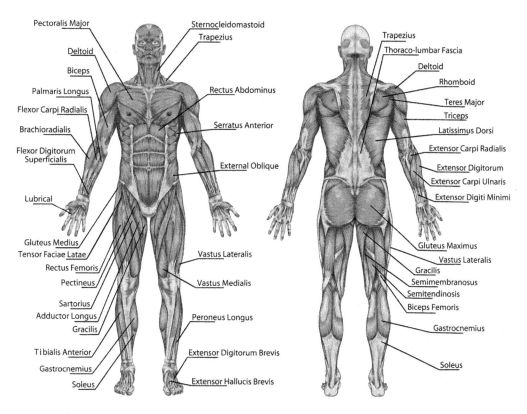

Figure 2.1 Anatomy of male muscular system – posterior and anterior view – full body – didactic.

DOI: 10.4324/9781003104803-2

Muscle Tissue

Skeletal

Striated in appearance and controlled by the somatic nervous system, skeletal muscle tissue consists of a bundle of muscle fibres, namely fascicule. These fascicules are cylindrical in shape and are surrounded by another protective covering formed from collagen. These fibres are then protected by another layer called the endomysium.

Smooth

Smooth muscle is classified as tonic or phasic and exhibits various patterns of electrical and mechanical activities (Feher, 2017). It does not have clearly visible striation on the cells and is found in the digestive tract and blood vessels where it helps to create stability and aid movement along these passages. Smooth muscle is involuntary and is controlled by the autonomic nervous system.

Cardiac

Found in the heart, cardiac muscle contracts to create the heartbeats and pump blood around the body. It is involuntary and controlled by the autonomous nervous system. Cardiac muscle cells appear striated or striped under a microscope, which occurs due to alternating filaments comprising of myosin and actin proteins. The darker stripes indicate thick filaments comprising of myosin proteins with the thinner, lighter filaments containing actin.

Structure of Skeletal Muscle

The structure of skeletal muscle is shown in Figure 2.2.
    Muscle tissue has four main properties:

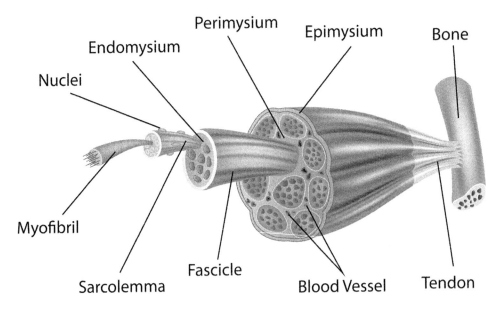

Figure 2.2 Illustration of structure skeletal muscle anatomy.

- Excitability – the ability to respond to a stimulus.
- Contractibility – the ability to contract.
- Extensibility – the ability to be lengthened without tearing.
- Elasticity – the ability to return to its original length following being stretched.

Muscle movements are defined as:

- Concentric – muscle generates force and shortens – lifting a weight up against gravity.
- Eccentric – muscle generates force and lengthens – lowering a weight down.
- Isometric – generates force – muscle length remains the same – holding a weight in the same position.

In summary, Wisdom et al. (2015) specified muscle force as *isometric* if generated by a muscle maintained at constant length; as *concentric* if generated through muscle shortening; and as *eccentric* if generated through muscle lengthening. When the sarcomeres operate at their optimal length, they generate maximum force. Peak isometric muscle stress refers to the maximum isometric muscle force divided by the physiological cross-sectional area of the whole muscle. Peak isometric fibre stress refers to the maximum isometric fibre force divided by the fibre cross-sectional area.

How Muscle Contracts

THE SLIDING FILAMENT THEORY – HUXLEY AND NIEDERGERKE (1954) AND HUXLEY AND HANSON (1954)

The sliding filament theory is described as follows: a nervous impulse arrives at the neuro-muscular junction. This causes a release of acetylcholine which leads to depolarisation of the motor end plate. Calcium is then released into the sarcoplasmic reticulum. These high levels of calcium bind to troponin, changing its shape to tropomyosin. Myosin can then attach to the actin forming a cross-bridging system (see Figure 2.3). The organic chemical adenosine triphosphate (ATP) is broken down, which releases energy enabling the myosin to pull the actin filaments, making the muscle shorten. As the myosin detaches from the actin, the cross-bridge is broken as the ATP molecule binds to the myosin head. Once ATP is again broken down it can again attach to an actin binding site further along the actin filament. The repeated 'pulling' motion of the actin over the myosin filaments is known as the 'ratchet' mechanism. As long as there is an adequate supply of ATP and calcium this process of muscular contraction is able to continue.

Although the sliding filament theory is still taught today, other theories have been proposed. Mungal and colleagues (2015) suggested that Z discs and actin filaments in the half part of each sarcomere, which is towards the origin end of muscle fibre, are not pulled toward the centre of the myosin filament; instead the myosin filament slides towards the origin end. And in the other half of each sarcomere (which is toward the insertion end), actin filaments slide over the myosin filament towards the origin end of the muscle. In addition, Herzog et al. (2016), based on their experimental observations and theoretical support, proposed that at least one of these structural proteins, titin, also contributes to 'active' force production; they proposed that titin changes its stiffness and force by binding calcium at specific sites, and by attaching to actin upon muscle activation and force production. The authors went

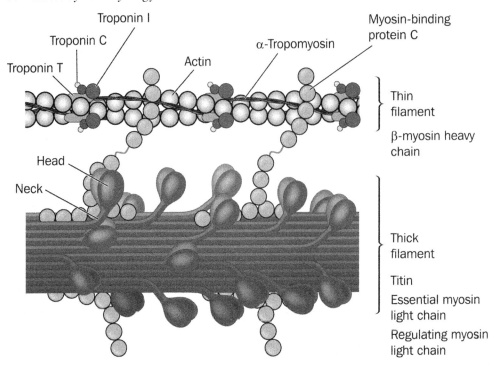

Figure 2.3 Detail of muscle tissue showing actin and myosin, troponin complex, thin filaments and thick filaments.

on to summarise the proposed action of titin in the new three-filament model of muscle contraction, in conjunction with the actin-myosin-based cross-bridge theory which could predict many basic properties of skeletal muscle contraction. Edman (2012) also noted that classic cross-bridge models cannot predict the residual force enhancement property, but residual force enhancement is a well-acknowledged and generally accepted property of skeletal muscles.

The Viscoelastic Properties of Muscle

Muscle and tendons are able to 'displace' under load. This stress and strain on the tissues is known as 'creep'. When the tissue is held at a constant strain level, the stress in the tissue decreases, a phenomenon called 'stress relaxation'. Muscles dissipate energy when they actively lengthen, and energy dissipation is required for any activity involving the deceleration of the body or limbs, including quick manoeuvres, reducing speed in walking or running, or landing from a jump (Roberts & Konow, 2013). Slow recovery after loading means a tendon is unlikely to achieve full recovery prior to subsequent loading and will deform more (from its original length) under similar loads (in creep scenarios); failure to recover completely from a stress relaxation scenario results in a slightly longer tendon, reducing the efficiency of the muscle-tendon contraction (Duenwald et al., 2009). The reduction in muscle lengthening is due to tendon elasticity and might serve a protective effect against muscle damage (tendon buffering). However, tendons dissipate only a small fraction (< 10%) of the energy they absorb, and the 'shock' they absorb at impact must eventually be released to the muscle, which dissipates the energy (Roberts & Konow, 2013).

Muscle Fibre Types

Type I muscle fibres (slow twitch) have a higher oxidative capacity and a higher fatigue threshold, firing more slowly than type II fibres, and are more suited to endurance sports. The high rate of protein turnover present in type I muscle fibres reflects the high adaptive potential of the tissue (Grgic et al., 2018). They are capable of producing repeated low-level contractions by producing large amounts of adenosine triphosphate (ATP).

Type II muscle fibres have faster calcium kinetics, faster shortening velocities, and the ability to generate more power than type I muscle fibres. Therefore, they are more suited to strength and speed-based sports and are classified as type IIa and IIb fibres.

Type IIa fibres use aerobic and anaerobic metabolism. They are a combination of type I and type II fibres. Type IIb fibres fire rapidly producing fast powerful bursts of speed, but they are also fast to fatigue. They produce ATP at a slower rate and break it down quickly.

When the muscle is at its resting length, the two sets of collagen fibres are arranged at angles of approximately 55° to the long axis of the muscle fibres. In other muscles, and especially in pennate muscles, the arrangement of collagen fibres in the epimysium is parallel to the long axis of the muscle and forms a dense surface layer that functions as a surface tendon (see the later section on ligaments and tendons). The perimysium is a continuous network of connective tissue which divides the muscle up into fascicles or muscle fibre bundles (Purslow, 2010).

Bones and Joints

The major bones of the human body are shown in Figure 2.4 and Table 2.1.

Bones consist of cells embedded in an abundant hard intercellular material. They are made from two principal components, collagen and calcium phosphate. Bones have a number of functions, which include structural support, protection of soft organs and tissues, providing an environment for bone marrow, acting as a storage area for minerals, and enabling the endocrine system to regulate the level of calcium and phosphate in circulating body fluids.

Calcium phosphate hardens the bone's framework, giving it its strength. More than 99% of our body's calcium is held in our bones and teeth, which have an internal structure similar to a honeycomb that makes them rigid but relatively light (Figure 2.5).

- Osteoblasts form new bone. They also originate from bone marrow and only have one cell. They produce new bone called 'osteoid', which is made from collagen and other proteins, and control the amount of calcium and minerals deposited. They line the surface of bones and fill cavities.
- Osteocytes are inside bone and come from inactive osteoblasts. Osteocytes originate from osteoblasts that have migrated into and become trapped and surrounded by bone matrix. They send out long branches that connect to the other osteocytes which sense pressures or cracks in the bone and help to direct where osteoclasts will dissolve the bone.
- Osteoclasts are very large multinucleate cells that are responsible for the breakdown of bones by the process of bone resorption. They degrade bone to initiate normal bone remodelling and mediate bone loss in pathologic conditions by increasing their resorptive activity. They regulate the differentiation of osteoblast precursors and the movement of

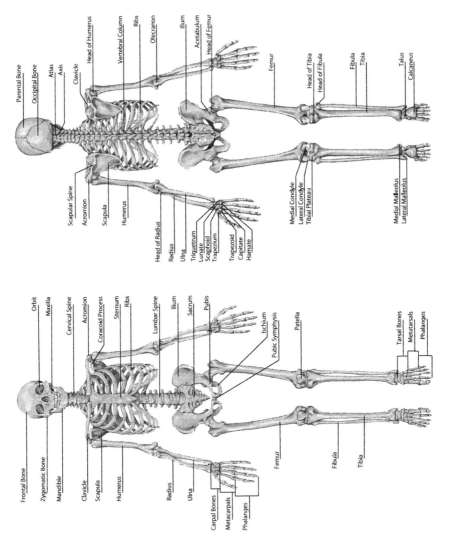

Figure 2.4 Major bones of the skeleton.

Table 2.1 The bones of the human body

Axial skeleton
Cranium	8 bones
Face	14 bones
Vertebral column	
Cervical	7 bones
Thoracic	12 bones
Lumbar	5 bones
Sacrum	5 bones (fused)
Coccyx	4 bones (fused)
Thorax	
Sternum	1 bone
Ribs	24 bones
Appendicular skeleton	
Clavicle	2 bones
Scapula	2 bones
Upper limb	
Humerus	2 bones
Ulna	2 bones
Radius	2 bones
Carpals	16 bones
Metacarpals	10 bones
Phalanges	28 bones
Pelvic (hip girdle)	
Coxal pelvis or hipbone	2 bones
Lower limbs	
Femur	2 bones
Fibula	2 bones
Tibia	2 bones
Patella	2 bones
Tarsals	14 bones
Metatarsals	10 bones
Phalanges	28 bones

hematopoietic stem cells from the bone marrow to the bloodstream; they participate in immune response and secrete cytokines that can affect their own functions and those of other cells in inflammatory and neoplastic processes affecting bone.

There are five types of bones in the skeleton: flat, long, short, sesamoid and irregular (mixed) (Figure 2.6).

Long bones, as the name suggests, are some of the longest bones in the body, including the femur, humerus and tibia. However, they are also some of the smallest, including the metacarpals, metatarsals, and phalanges. This is due to their classification, which includes having a body which is longer than it is wide, with growth plates (epiphysis) at either end; having a hard-outer surface of a compact bone and a spongy inner layer, known as cancellous bone; and containing bone marrow. They are also lined with hyaline cartilage.

Flat or cuboidal bones are the same width and length and have flat plates, with the main function of providing protection to the body's vital organs and being a base for muscular attachment. Examples include the scapula (shoulder blade), the sternum (breastbone), ilium (hip bone), pelvis and ribs. Anterior and posterior surfaces are formed of compact bone to

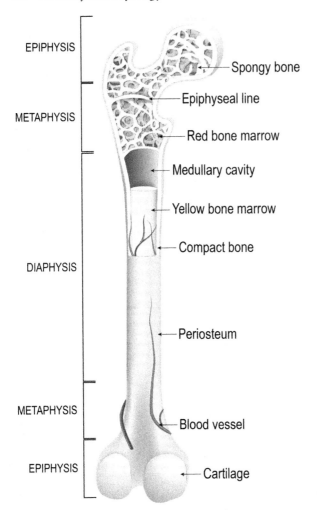

EPIPHYSIS

METAPHYSIS

DIAPHYSIS

METAPHYSIS

EPIPHYSIS

Spongy bone

Epiphyseal line

Red bone marrow

Medullary cavity

Yellow bone marrow

Compact bone

Periosteum

Blood vessel

Cartilage

Figure 2.5 Bone anatomy.

provide strength for protection with the centre consisting of cancellous (spongy) bone and varying amounts of bone marrow. In adults, they also contain red blood cells.

Irregular (mixed) bones are bones with complex shapes. These bones may have short, flat, notched, or ridged surfaces; for example, the vertebrae, hip bones, and several skull bones. They help protect internal organs, for example, the vertebrae protect the spinal cord and the pelvis protects the organs in the pelvic cavity.

Sesamoid bones are small flat bones, for example the patella. Sesamoid bones develop inside tendons and may be found near joints at the knees, hands, and feet.

Joints

The point at which two or more bones meet is called a joint, or articulation. Joints are responsible for movement and provide stability.

Joints are classified by their structure or their function.

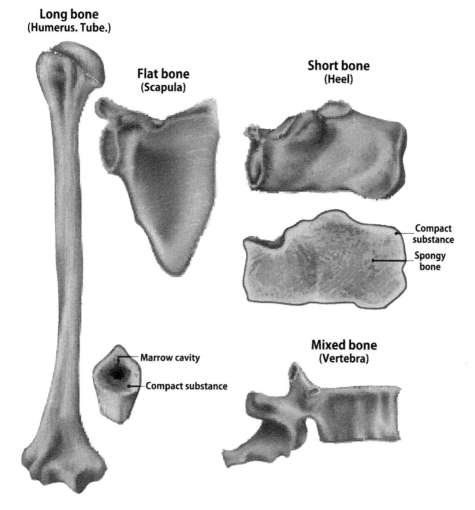

Long bone
(Humerus. Tube.)

Flat bone
(Scapula)

Short bone
(Heel)

Compact
substance

Spongy
bone

Marrow cavity

Compact substance

Mixed bone
(Vertebra)

Figure 2.6 Types of bones.

Joint Structures

Fibrous joints are held together by fibrous connective tissue. There is no cavity between the structure, therefore there is very little movement. The three types of fibrous joints are syndesmoses, gomphoses and sutures. Sutures are only found in the skull; syndesmoses are connected by a band of connective tissue, for example in the tibia and fibula joint. Gomphoses refers to the way the teeth fit into the socket (by connective tissue called the periodontal ligament).

SYNOVIAL JOINTS

Synovial joints comprise a fibrous capsule surrounded by ligaments that link the bones and provide stability. For example, the strength of the knee is determined by the anterior and posterior cruciate ligaments and the medial and lateral collateral ligaments. The hip (ball and socket joint) is formed with the head of the femur fitting neatly into the socket (acetabulum) in the pelvis.

CARTILAGE

Cartilage is a connective tissue made up of specialized cells called chondrocytes which produce large amounts of extracellular matrix, which is composed of collagen fibres, proteoglycan and elastin fibres.

Articular (hyaline) cartilage bears and distributes weight and is flexible. It reduces friction but has a poor blood supply. It covers and protects the ends of the bones where they meet to form a joint.

Fibrocartilage is tough and inflexible. It contains many bundles of collagenous fibres and gives strength and rigidity to, for example, the menisci in the knee and the intervertebral discs in the spine. Fibroelastic cartilage combines strength and elasticity for structures such as the ear, the epiglottis and the larynx. It can change its shape in response to tension and compression and has the ability to snap back to its original form, providing a flexible but strong structure.

Anatomical Positions and Movement

Axes and Planes

There are three planes and associated axes of the body (Figure 2.7). The sagittal (lateral) plane divides the body into left and right. The frontal (coronal) plane is the vertical plane that lies at right angles to both the median and the frontal plane and divides the body into front and back halves or anterior and posterior portions. The transverse or axial (horizontal) plane passes at right angles to both the median and the frontal planes and divides the body into upper and lower parts (head and tail portions).

The anatomical terms for describing positions of parts of the body:

- Medial – nearer to the median plane.
- Lateral – further away from the median plane.
- Proximal – nearer to the point of attachment of a limb to the trunk.
- Distal – further from the point of attachment of a limb to the trunk.
- Anterior (ventral) – towards the front of the body.
- Posterior (dorsal) – towards the back of the body.
- Inferior – closer to the feet.
- Superior – closer to the head.
- Supine – describes the position of a body lying horizontal and face up.
- Prone – describes the position of a body lying horizontal and face down.

Movements

The anatomical terms for describing movements of the body are listed below.

- Flexion – a reduction in the angle between bones at a joint, i.e. bending the joint.
- Extension – an increase in the angle between bones at a joint, i.e. straightening the joint.
- Abduction – movement of a limb away from the median plane.
- Adduction – movement of a limb towards the median plane.
- Circumduction – a circular limb movement which combines in sequence flexion, extension, abduction and adduction.

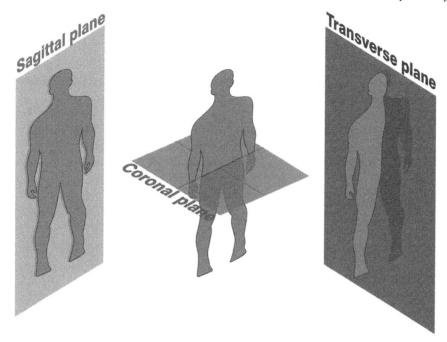

Figure 2.7 Vector illustration of anatomical planes of body section.

- Rotation – movement of a limb around its long axis. Medial rotation turns the anterior surface medially, and lateral rotation turns it laterally.
- Dorsiflexion – movement of the foot to point the toes upwards.
- Plantarflexion – movement of the foot to point the toes downwards.
- Protraction – draws the shoulder girdle forwards around the chest wall.
- Retraction – draws the shoulder girdle backwards around the chest wall, so the shoulders are 'braced' as in a military stance.
- Elevation – lifts the scapula upwards, as in shrugging the shoulders.
- Depression – drops the scapula downwards to lower the shoulders.
- Supination – a rotary movement of the forearm so the palm faces upwards.
- Pronation – a rotary movement of the forearm so the palm faces downwards. The terms pronation and supination are also used in reference to the foot, i.e. a pronated foot, meaning a flat foot.
- Inversion – turns the sole of the foot inwards.
- Eversion – turns the sole of the foot outwards.
- Lateral flexion – bends the trunk in the frontal plane (see above).
- Contralateral – to the symmetrically opposite side
- Ipsilateral – to the same side.

Ligaments and Tendons

Ligaments

The primary fibrous constituent of ligament is type I collagen, a structural protein that assembles hierarchically from tropocollagen into fibrils, fibres and then fascicles. Collagen networks in healthy ligament, as well as tendon, typically exhibit uniaxial alignment (Stender et al., 2018). They are defined as dense bands of collagenous tissue (fibres) that span a joint and then become anchored to the bone at either end (Frank, 2004). Although ligaments are similar in structure to tendons, they have a higher proteoglycan matrix than tendons and their collagen fibrils are slightly less in volume fraction and organisation. Ligaments often have a more vascular overlying layer termed the 'epiligament' covering their surface, and this layer is often indistinguishable from the actual ligament (Frank, 2004).

Tendons

Tendons are a connective tissue that attach muscle to bone. They are primarily made of type I collagen with the remaining 20–30% of dry weight coming from proteoglycans, glycosaminoglycans, type III, IV, V, XII and elastin (Tresoldi et al., 2013), which enables them to withstand high forces when transferring loads between tissues (McCarthy & Hannafin, 2014; Connizzo et al., 2015). They are able to resist both tensile and compressive stress due to the direction of their fibre orientation and proteoglycan content. Tendons generally have a good blood supply which they receive from the musculotendinous junction, the osseo-tendinous junction, and the surrounding soft tissues (McCarthy & Hannafin, 2014).

Skin

The skin is a complex heterogeneous adaptive structure (Figure 2.8) which varies according to body location, health status and history, diet, age, lifestyle, *external* environmental conditions

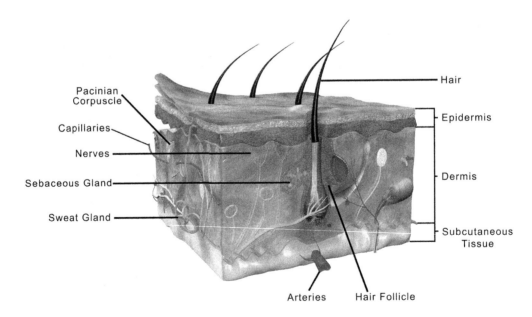

Figure 2.8 Skin anatomy 3D illustration.

(e.g. temperature, humidity, pollution level, water quality, sun exposure, contact with external surfaces) and *internal* environmental conditions (e.g. hormones, pregnancy, water and glucose levels, tension lines). Besides intra-individual variability, there is a strong biophysical variability, particularly that associated with sex and ethnicity (Limbert, 2017).

It is the largest organ in the human body, yet its importance in maintaining homeostasis, providing us with sensory feedback, and protecting us against our environment is frequently overlooked. The top layer is the epidermis, the second layer is the dermis (the dermis and the epidermis together are also referred to as cutis) and the third layer is the hypodermis (subcutaneous tissue). The dermis is a moderately dense connective tissue which comprises three fibrous proteins – collagen, elastin, and minute quantities of reticulin – and a supporting matrix or ground substance. Among the extracellular matrix molecules in the dermis, versican appears to be the most important molecule for tissue viscoelasticity (and subcutaneous tissues) which gradually decreases with age, leading to a reduction of viscoelasticity (Nemoto et al., 2012).

Skin viscoelasticity incorporates the water content of the skin (20%) and adds the principle of viscosity, the internal resistance to flow when a shearing force or stress is applied to a fluid. Hyaluronic acid absorbs water, forming a thick gel that impedes the bulk flow of fluid and creates hydrostatic pressure and skin turgor; the hydrostatic pressure resists compressive forces, protects the solid structures of the skin, and contributes to its viscoelastic behaviour (Everet & Sommers, 2013). As a result of its viscoelastic properties, skin is able to deform and 'creep'. Mechanical creep is the elongation of skin with a constant load over time beyond intrinsic extensibility. Creep deformation does not occur suddenly at the application of stress; instead, strain accumulates as a result of long-term stress. To summarise Holzapfel's (2001) comprehensive paper on the biomechanics of soft tissue, the deformation behaviour for skin may be studied in three phases (I, II and III). Initially, low stress is required to achieve large deformations of the individual collagen fibres without requiring stretch of the fibres. The stress-strain relation is approximately linear, the elastic modulus of skin in phase I is low (0.1–2 MPa). In phase II, as the load is increased, the collagen fibres tend to line up with the load direction and bear loads. The crimped collagen fibres gradually elongate. With deformation the crimp angle in collagen fibrils leads to a sequential uncrimping of fibrils. In phase III, at high tensile stresses, the crimp patterns disappear and the collagen fibers become straighter. They are primarily aligned with one another in the direction in which the load is applied. The straightened collagen fibers resist the load strongly and the tissue becomes stiff at higher stresses. Beyond the third phase the ultimate tensile strength is reached and fibers begin to break

In conclusion, the skin has a number of important roles. They include protecting the body from the external physical and chemical environment, regulating temperature via vasodilation or vasoconstriction of blood vessels, the excretion of sweat and providing sensation (pressure, touch and pain).

Fascia

Before we can determine if massage, foam rolling and instrument-assisted therapy tools have an effect on fascia, we have to understand what fascia actually is. Shah and Bhalara (2012) described it as 'the underlying structure of muscle and bone, it is a seamless web of connective tissue that covers and connects the muscles, organs, and skeletal structures in our body'. At the 4th International Fascia Research Congress, Stecco and Schleip (2016) declared 'fascia is a sheath, a sheet, or any number of other dissectible aggregations of connective tissue that forms beneath the skin to attach, enclose, and separate muscles and other internal organs'. Recently, Bordoni and Meyers (2020) reported the latest definition of fascia (2019): fascia is any tissue that contains features capable of responding to mechanical stimuli. The fascial continuum is the result of the evolution of the perfect synergy among different tissues, liquids and solids, capable of supporting, dividing, penetrating, feeding and connecting all the regions of the body, from the epidermis to the bone, involving all its functions and organic structures. This continuum constantly transmits and receives mechano-metabolic information that can influence the shape and function of the entire body. These afferent/efferent impulses come from the fascia and the tissues that are not considered part of the fascia in a biunivocal mode. In this definition, these tissues include 'epidermis, dermis, fat, blood, lymph, and lymphatic vessels, tissue covering the nervous filaments (endoneurium, perineurium, epineurium), voluntary striated muscle fibres and the tissue covering and permeating it (epimysium, perimysium, endomysium), ligaments, tendons, aponeurosis, cartilage, bones, meninges, and tongue' (Bordoni et al., 2019).

Fascia is a connective tissue composed of irregularly arranged collagen fibres embedded in a gelatinous ground substance (Standring, 2008). This ground substance has a gel-like consistency similar to raw egg white which reduces friction between muscle fibres, creating ease of motion (Shah & Bhalara, 2012). It has been hypothesised any impediment to gliding between endofascial fibres and interfascial planes could cause anomalous tension, and given that many mechanoreceptors are embedded within fascia, altered proprioceptive afferents could then result in non-physiologic movements at joints (Stecco & Day, 2010). Such movements could cause inflammation within the joint of a malfunctioning myofascial unit, or pain along a myofascial sequence (Stecco & Day, 2010).

Fascia assumes a fundamental role with its two components: dense connective tissue (collagen fibres type I and III) and loose connective tissue (adipose cells, glycosaminoglycans [GAGs] and hyaluronan [HA]) (Cowman et al., 2015). It contains four types of sensory nerve endings, which are responsive to mechanical stimulation: Golgi organs, Ruffini receptors, Pacini corpuscles and interstitial receptors. It is known that the HA is one of the most important elements that determines the viscoelasticity of a tissue. Its important presence inside the fascia could permit us to suppose that its alteration could modify the activation of the receptors inside the fascia. This could be the origin of the common phenomenon of myofascial pain (Stecco et al., 2011).

Fascial tissues are commonly used as elastic springs (catapult action) during oscillatory movements, such as walking, hopping, or running, in which the supporting skeletal muscles contract rather isometrically and are prone to viscoelastic deformations such as creep, hysteresis and relaxation. Such temporary deformations alter fascial stiffness and may take several hours for recovery (Schleip et al., 2010). In addition, it is also worth noting fascia thickness differs substantially between older and younger individuals exhibiting regional specialisations: while younger people have a thicker connective tissue in the lower limb, elderly individuals display a higher fascial thickness in the low back region (Wilke et al., 2019). Therefore, understanding that certain types of fascia are more densely populated with certain particular receptors can aid in the overall understanding of the body and creating more effective approaches to manual treatments (Kumka & Bonar, 2012). Myofascial release techniques are explained in Chapter 5 and in the first section of Chapter 11, on foam rolling.

The Lymphatic System

Lymph nodes are especially fascinating organs that provide a specialised microenvironment for the meeting of migratory immune cells, especially lymphocytes and antigen-presenting cells like dendritic cells (DCs) (Randolph et al., 2017). The lymphatic system (Figure 2.9) has been identified to actively regulate numerous physiological and pathological processes (Aspelund et al., 2016) and acts as a passive transit system from the extracellular space to the blood circulation by using an active pump-based mechanism to export interstitial fluid and its

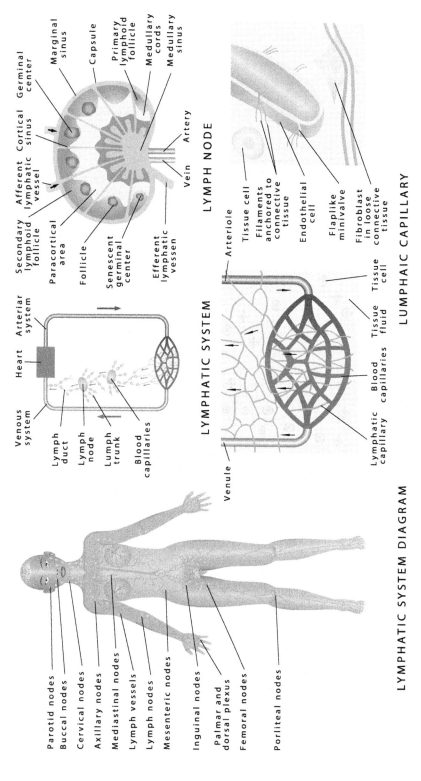

Figure 2.9 Lymphatic system.

contents directly out of tissue (Randolph et al., 2017). Unlike the blood vessels in the circulatory system, lymphatic vessels are blind-ended unidirectional absorptive vessels, transporting interstitial fluid, immune cells and macromolecules to the lymph nodes (LNs) and back to the blood circulation, which actively overcome net pressure gradients (Aspelund et al., 2016) of approximately 20 cmH$_2$O (Moore & Bertram, 2018). To do so, the collecting vessels contain intraluminal valves to prevent backflow and are covered by smooth muscle cells, which periodically contract to drive lymph forward. In addition, extrinsic compression by the surrounding tissue during muscle activity significantly contributes to lymph propulsion (Aspelund et al., 2016).

Following injury, the inflammatory process follows, and a number of events take place, starting with bleeding, leading to fluid accumulation into the intercellular spaces and the formation of oedema. Once oedema has formed, the lymphatic system plays a role in removing excess interstitial fluid and returning the fluid to the circulatory system. Despite anecdotal claims, Vairo et al.'s (2009) systematic review of literature concluded that the influence of manual lymphatic drainage techniques for specific conditions encountered in conventional athletic injury rehabilitation is limited, and is founded upon hypotheses, theory and preliminary evidence.

Manual therapy stimulates the lymphatic system via an increase in lymph circulation, by expediting the removal of biochemical wastes from body tissues. It enhances body fluid dynamics, thereby facilitating oedema reduction, and decreases sympathetic nervous system responses while increasing parasympathetic nervous tone (Vairo et al., 2009). This was described in greater detail by Majewski-Schrage and Snyder (2016) in their article on the manual lymphatic drainage treatment process in patients with orthopaedic injuries. The authors reported that firstly, treatment is initiated through proximal pre-treatment by emptying the truncal regions to stimulate lymphangion activity, removing static fluid, and ultimately allowing distal fluid to be transferred through the lymph vessels. Secondly, subsequent extremity-specific massage is commenced. The proximal region is cleared first, working distally to push lymph into emptied proximal regions. Thirdly, strokes are applied with very light pressure, allowing the skin to slightly stretch rather than simply sliding over the surface. A pumping effect is achieved through two different stroke phases. And finally, a thrust phase is followed by a relaxation phase.

Eighteen healthy male volunteers were subjected to a graded exercise test by Bakar and colleagues (2015) to assess the effects of manual lymphatic drainage massage on lactate clearance and muscle damage. Following sub-maximal exercise, manual lymphatic drainage correlated with a more rapid fall in lactic acid, lactate dehydrogenase, creatine kinase, and myoglobin, and may result in improvements in the regeneration process following exercise, allowing the vessels to accumulate fluid. In their study the authors also concluded that due to the lack of homogeneity between studies, manual lymphatic drainage (MLD) was not superior compared to no treatment; however, it may help decrease oedema and increase range of motion and activities of living. In 50 women with fibromyalgia receiving either manual lymphatic drainage or connective tissue massage, Ekici et al. (2009) found both groups had significant improvements in pain intensity and health-related quality of life scores; however, manual lymphatic drainage was preferred, according to some subitems of the fibromyalgia impact questionnaire (FIQ) (morning tiredness and anxiety and FIQ total score).

Contraindications to lymphatic drainage massage include major cardiac pathologies, thrombosis or venous obstruction, haemorrhage, acute enuresis and malignant tumours.

Blood

Blood cell types are shown in Figure 2.10.

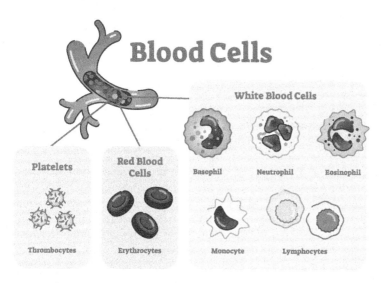

Figure 2.10 Blood cells.

- Erythrocytes – red blood cells. Red blood cells are produced in the soft red bone marrow and make up approximately 40% of the total blood volume. Haemoglobin in red blood cells binds to oxygen, allowing the transportation of oxygen and carbon dioxide around the body. Checking the number of erythrocytes in the blood is usually part of a complete blood cell (CBC) test and may be used to look for conditions such as anaemia, dehydration, malnutrition and leukaemia.
- Leukocytes – white blood cells. There are approximately 700 times fewer white blood cells than red blood cells. They are produced in the soft red bone marrow. They form an integral part of natural defence against infections and pathogens by destroying bacteria and provide immunity to the body.
- Thrombocytes – platelets. Platelets are cell fragments (averaging about 2–4um in diameter) which helps to promote blood clotting at the site of any damaged tissues. The function of the platelets is to prevent and control bleeding. When the endothelial surface (lining) of a blood vessel is injured, platelets immediately attach to the injured surface and to each other, forming a larger group of platelets to develop a blood clot.
- Plasma – the liquid portion of blood; it consists of 91.5% water and 8.5% solutes (including proteins, electrolytes, nutrients, gases and hormones), and comprises about 55% of blood's overall content. The role of plasma is to transport nutrients, hormones and proteins to the parts of the body that need it.

Soft Tissue Injury and Stages of Healing

When a soft tissue injury occurs, the aim for the sports massage therapist, alongside other members of the sports and exercise medicine team, is to promote healing, break the pain-injury cycle, return the athlete to their pre-injury state and prevent re-injury occurring, all in the shortest time frame possible. This means throughout the healing process the athlete needs to maintain rest-of-body conditioning in order to maintain fitness levels.

When a muscle is exposed to an excessive extrinsic tensile force that induces muscle shearing a 'strain' will occur. This exercise-induced muscle injury will cause swelling and an intramuscular haematoma. Blood within the intact muscle fascia increases intramuscular pressure, which subsequently compresses the bleeding blood vessels and thereby eventually limits the size of the haematoma. In a severe strain the epimysium of the injured muscle may also rupture and then an intermuscular hematoma develops (Järvinen et al., 2013).

Muscle injuries are common in all sports, and for example in soccer, they account for 31% of all injuries (Ekstrand et al., 2011). They usually occur during the eccentric phase of muscle contraction and predominately affect muscles with a higher percentage of type II fibres and those that cross two joints and have a pennate architecture, for example, hamstrings and rectus femoris.

Traditionally muscle injuries have been graded between I and III depending on their severity. A mild (grade I) strain usually presents as a tear of only a few muscle fibres with minor swelling and discomfort, accompanied with no or only minimal loss of strength and restrictions during movement. A moderate (grade II) strain has greater damage of the muscle with a clear loss of function. Severe (grade III) strains occur when a tear extends across the entire cross-section of the muscle and usually results in complete loss of muscle function. However, a study involving 207 elite European footballers failed to show a statistically significant difference in prognosis between grade I and II injuries (Ekstrand et al., 2012), highlighting that a bad grade I is very similar to a moderate grade II. In reality the treatment and rehabilitation protocol would be the same, or very similar for the majority of grade I and II injuries and should only be considered a guide for the therapist. In fact, it is now recommended structural injuries are based on anatomical findings. In addition to the size, it is the participation of the adjacent connective tissue, the endomysium, the perimysium, the epimysium and the fascia that distinguish a minor from a moderate partial muscle tear (Meuller-Wohlfahrt et al., 2013).

Wilke and colleagues (2019) made an important point in their systematic review and meta-analysis of the prevalence of extra-muscular connective tissue lesions in muscle strain injury. The authors found isolated muscular lesions were identified only in about one of eight cases, and the damage was frequently located within or at the junction to the collagenous connective tissue. The term 'muscle strain injury' therefore, does not adequately reflect the morphological substrate of the condition and could be misleading during the diagnostic process. To avoid this, the authors suggested using more general terms (e.g. 'myo-collagenous strain injury') that may indicate more clearly the variety of potentially affected tissues.

Stages of Healing

During the acute phase, previously the acronym *PRICE* (protection, rest, ice, compression and elevation) has been used, despite a paucity of high-quality, empirical evidence to support the various components, or as a collective treatment package (Bleakley et al., 2012). Another acronym, *POLICE*, which represents protection, optimal loading, ice compression and elevation, has also been used, stressing the importance of early 'optimal' loading:

Protection of the injured area from further damage by monitoring external symptoms and avoiding excessive loading.

Optimal loading is engaging in early, controlled movement by limiting (and gradually increasing) the workload as physiological capacity is restored. This may include the use of crunches to encourage partial weight bearing and gait re-education, the alter-G (anti-gravity treadmill) or hydrotherapy.

Ice should be applied for 15–20 minutes at a time within the first 48–72 hours of injury for its analgesic effect (pain gate theory).

Compression bandages can help minimize swelling, stop greater haemorrhage and prevent excessive movement.

Elevation of the injured area to limit blood pooling and assist in venous return.

The latest acronym to surface is *PEACE* and *LOVE* (Dubois & Esculier, 2020):

Protection – avoid activities that can increase pain during the first few days after injury. Rest should be minimised as prolonged rest can compromise tissue strength and quality.

Elevation – elevate the limb higher than the heart to promote interstitial fluid flow out of the tissue.

Avoid anti-inflammatories – anti-inflammatory medications may potentially be detrimental for long-term tissue healing.

Compression – external mechanical pressure using taping or bandages helps to limit intra-articular oedema and tissue haemorrhage.

Education – therapists should educate patients on the benefits of an active approach to recovery.

Load – movement and exercise will benefit most athletes with musculoskeletal disorders. Mechanical stress should be added early, and normal activities resumed as soon as pain/symptoms allow. Optimal loading without exacerbating pain promotes repair, remodelling and building tissue tolerance and capacity of tendons, muscles and ligaments through mechano-transduction.

Optimism – the brain plays a key role in rehabilitation interventions. Psychological factors such as catastrophising, depression and fear can represent barriers to recovery. While staying realistic, practitioners should encourage optimism to enhance the likelihood of optimal recovery.

Vascularisation – pain-free physical activity that includes cardiovascular components should be started a few days after injury to boost motivation and increase blood flow to the injured structures.

Exercise – exercises will help to restore mobility, strength, and proprioception early after injury.

The acronyms may change in sports medicine; however, athletes do not have 'time' for normal tissue healing to take place due to competition schedules or forthcoming matches, so they will look to bypass many of the *PEACE* and *LOVE* phases. For example, the use of injection therapy and tight strapping in order to compete is a common occurrence.

Sub-Acute Stage

Regeneration now begins. At the early stage of muscle regeneration, the injured muscle cells undergo necrosis in response to trauma. The blood contains inflammatory cells that infiltrate the newly injured area (neutrophils, lymphoid cells, B cells, T cells, epithelial cells, stem cells). During the repair stage macrophages 'eat' and clean away any dead tissue. A satellite cell is then released transforming into myoblast cells which come together to create new muscle fibres. Another new cell, fibroblasts, build connective and muscle tissue. Remodelling now takes place as muscle and connective tissue mature into the final scar tissue. It is at this time the therapist can have the greatest input by making sure the fibres are organised in straight lines rather than a disorganised clump of fibres (adhesions).

In this phase, treatment options include massage (effleurage and light petrissage techniques) and contrast therapy for pain gate and circulation. Gentle stretching and mobility exercises can be implemented to discourage neuromuscular adhesions. During the later stages of this phase, easy proprioception exercises, correct gait education and low load isometric exercises can be encouraged in conjunction with a rest-of-body workout.

Post Sub-Acute Phase

The treatment and exercises can now be advanced to prepare the athlete for return to play/competition, with massage and stretching intensity and duration increased. Movement patterns can become more complex, encouraging multi-joint, multi-muscle movements leading to specific patterns from the athlete's sport. The injured limb should have gradually increased loads in the isometric, eccentric and concentric phases of the selected exercise. Proprioception should be increased using unstable surfaces, increased loads and more challenging movements should be encouraged.

Fractures

When bone receives too much force it can break. There are a number of types of fracture which can occur (see Figure 2.11). When bone fragments stick out through the skin, or a wound penetrates down to the broken bone, the fracture is called an 'open' fracture. Once the skin is broken the bone is open to infection.

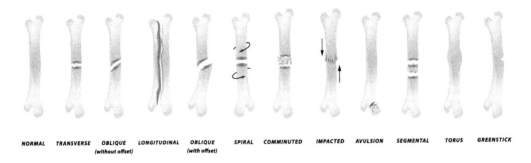

NORMAL   TRANSVERSE   OBLIQUE   LONGITUDINAL   OBLIQUE   SPIRAL   COMMINUTED   IMPACTED   AVULSION   SEGMENTAL   TORUS   GREENSTICK
(without offset)   (with offset)

Figure 2.11 Types of fracture.

In the athletic population, fractures are usually a result of direct trauma, for example, in a tackle during a football game when an opponent hits the planted foot between the ankle and the knee. In the female athlete triad, a syndrome composed of the following three interrelated conditions: low energy availability, menstrual dysfunction and poor bone health, osteoporosis and stress fractures can occur (Mallinson & De Sousa, 2014). The International Olympic Committee (IOC) consensus statement (2014) commented 'the clinical phenomenon is not a "triad" of the three entities of energy availability, menstrual function and bone health, but rather a syndrome that affects many aspects of physiological function, health and athletic performance' (Mountjoy et al., 2014). Poor bone health in women with the female athlete triad is characterised by detrimental changes in bone density and structure which, ultimately, may lead to clinical endpoints such as osteoporosis and fractures. The prevalence of athletes who fall under the female athlete triad remains unknown; by the early definition (disordered eating, amenorrhea, and osteoporosis), studies showed 1–4% prevalence among female athletes (Brown et al., 2017).

Pain Gate Theory

Melzack & Wall's (1965) idea that physical pain is not a direct result of activation of pain receptor neurons, but rather its perception is modulated by interaction between different neurons, is still used to explain phantom and chronic pain. They believed there is a 'gating system' in the central nervous system that opens and closes to let pain messages through to the brain or to block them (Figure 2.12). Pain is a subjective experience mediated by a variety of physiological and psychological factors; however, there is no single prevailing theory of pain that explains its origin, qualities, and alleviation (Lang et al., 2020).

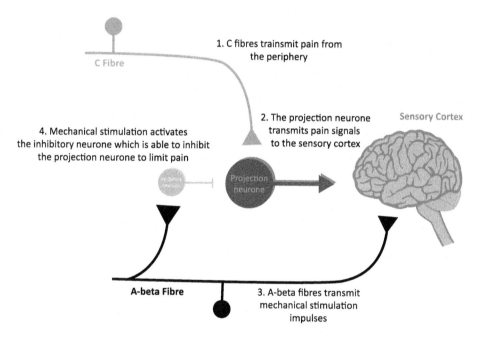

Figure 2.12 Gate control theory of pain illustration.

Nociceptors (free nerve endings) have a relatively high threshold to activation and are sensitive to potential tissue damage. Free nerve endings convey the action potential through the spinal cord.

A (Type III) fibres are involved in the withdrawal process (touching something hot), carry fast or transient pain and are myelinated.

C (Type IV) fibres are demyelinated, carry slow throbbing or prolonged pain, involve a greater degree of tissue damage and release chemical mediators i.e. bradykinin, histamine, prostaglandin, substance P and 5-HT. The withdrawal reflex and crossed extensor reflex happens once the nociceptor afferent enters the spinal cord via the dorsal root and makes synaptic connections. Presynaptic inhibition allows nociceptive information to be passed to a higher centre, through the thalamus and to the cerebral cortex. The pain gate theory argues that thoughts, beliefs and emotions affect the amount of pain felt from a given physical sensation and the way the individual responds to these sensations. Massage stimulates the mechanoreceptors in the skin (physiological effect) by the afferent signals blocking the pain transmission (pain gate theory) this with positive reinforcement, the perception of pain decreases (psychological effect).

It is quite plausible that massage can have both a physiological and psychological effect on pain, but there is a low strength of evidence due to the lack of primary studies of large sample sizes conducted with rigorous methods, leaving evidence gaps about specific massage type for specific pain. Primary studies often do not provide adequate details of massage therapy provided, limiting the extent to which reviews are able to draw conclusions about characteristics such as provider type (Miake-Lye et al., 2019).

Physiology of the Ageing Athlete

Over the course of an athlete's lifetime anatomy and physiology will change, due to the natural ageing process, continual micro-trauma from repetitive movements and loading, a result of direct impact (trauma), medication and drug use, and other non-sport related lifestyle choices. This said, masters or senior age grouped recreational and professional athletes are competing longer, with the list of available events growing year on year. For example, in 2018, John Starbrook completed his 33rd London Marathon aged 87. The Lawn Tennis Association has ranking listings (and competitions) for each age group from 35+ to 85+, and the British Masters Athletic Association holds events for a wide range of ages across a number of events (Figure 2.13).

In athletes over 40, higher injury rates generally occur as a result of changes within muscle, such as the re-arrangement of motor units and denervation. Even though the residual motor units will hypertrophy, their capacity to finely regulate force intensity will be lower

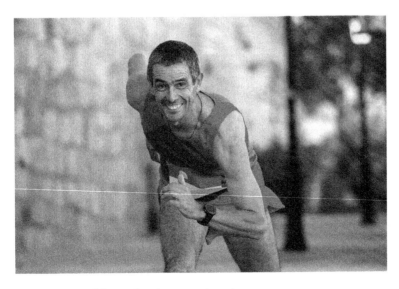

Figure 2.13 Middle-aged male runner in a city.

(Maffulli et al., 2015). The rate of muscle decline after 40 years of age has been shown to be about 0.5% to 1% per year (Paddon-Jones et al., 2008). The progressive loss of skeletal muscle mass and strength is a hallmark of the ageing process and is referred to as sarcopenia (Snijders et al., 2017) and is believed to be caused by a lack of tissue perfusion/oxygenation, the loss of alpha motoneurons, a reduction in plasma testosterone levels (particularly in the sixth decade), and growth hormone (GH) (after the third decade of life, there is a progressive decline of GH secretion by approximately 14–15% for every decade of adult life). In summary, this decline in strength and muscle mass is due to an overall loss of muscle tissue, and to a decrease in the proportion of type II fibres (Staunton et al., 2012). In addition, the tendons of veteran and master's series athletes have shown to have structural and compositional changes, including decreased water content, sectional hypo-vascularity, and collagenous changes (Weinreb et al., 2014), leading to higher injury rates than their younger counterparts.

References

Aspelund, A., Robciuc, M.R., Karaman, S., Makinen, T. and Alitalo, K., 2016. Lymphatic system in cardiovascular medicine. *Circulation Research*, 118(3), pp. 515–530.

Bakar, Y., Coknaz, H., Karlı, Ü., Semsek, Ö., Serın, E. and Pala, Ö.O., 2015. Effect of manual lymph drainage on removal of blood lactate after submaximal exercise. *Journal of Physical Therapy Science*, 27(11), pp. 3387–3391.

Bleakley, C.M., Glasgow, P. and MacAuley, D.C., 2012. PRICE needs updating, should we call the POLICE? *British Journal of Sports Medicine*, 46, pp. 220–221.

Bordoni, B. and Myers, T., 2020. A review of the theoretical fascial models: Biotensegrity, fascintegrity, and myofascial chains. *Cureus*, 12(2). doi: 10.1519/jsc.0000000000003395.

Bordoni, B., Simonelli, M. and Morabito, B., 2019. The other side of the fascia: The smooth muscle part 1. *Cureus*, 11(5): e4651. DOI 10.7759/cureus.4651.

Bordoni, B., Walkowski, S., Morabito, B. and Varacallo, M.A., 2019. Fascial nomenclature: An update. *Cureus*, 11(9). doi: 10.7759/cureus.4651.

Brown, K.A., Dewoolkar, A.V., Baker, N. and Dodich, C., 2017. The female athlete triad: Special considerations for adolescent female athletes. *Translational Pediatrics*, 6(3), p. 144.

Connizzo, B.K., Freedman, B.R., Fried, J.H., Sun, M., Birk, D.E. and Soslowsky, L.J., 2015. Regulatory role of collagen V in establishing mechanical properties of tendons and ligaments is tissue dependent. *Journal of Orthopaedic Research*, 33(6), pp. 882–888.

Cowman, M.K., Schmidt, T.A., Raghavan, P. and Stecco, A., 2015. Viscoelastic properties of hyaluronan in physiological conditions. *F1000Research*, 4, p. 622.

Dubois, B. and Esculier, J.F., 2020. Soft-tissue injuries simply need PEACE and LOVE. *Br Journal Sports Medicine*, 54(2), pp. 72–73. https://blogs.bmj.com/bjsm/2019/04/26/soft-tissue-injuries-simply-need-peace-love/

Duenwald, S.E., Vanderby, R. and Lakes, R.S., 2009. Viscoelastic relaxation and recovery of tendon. *Annals of Biomedical Engineering*, 37(6), pp. 1131–1140.

Edman, K.A.P., 2012. Residual force enhancement after stretch in striated muscle. A consequence of increased myofilament overlap? *The Journal of Physiology*, 590(6), pp. 1339–1345.

Ekici, G., Bakar, Y., Akbayrak, T. and Yuksel, I., 2009. Comparison of manual lymph drainage therapy and connective tissue massage in women with fibromyalgia: A randomized controlled trial. *Journal of Manipulative and Physiological Therapeutics*, 32(2), pp. 127–133.

Ekstrand, J., Hägglund, M. and Waldén, M., 2011. Epidemiology of muscle injuries in professional football (soccer). *The American Journal of Sports Medicine*, 39(6), pp. 1226–1232.

Ekstrand, J., Healy, J.C., Waldén, M., Lee, J.C., English, B. and Hägglund, M., 2012. Hamstring muscle injuries in professional Football: The correlation of MRI findings with return to play. *British Journal of Sports Medicine*, 46(2), pp. 112–117.

Everett, J.S. and Sommers, M.S., 2013. Skin viscoelasticity: Physiologic mechanisms, measurement issues, and application to nursing science. *Biological Research for Nursing*, *15*(3), pp. 338–346.

Feher, J.J., 2017. *Quantitative human physiology: An introduction*. Elsevier: Academic Press.

Frank, C.B., 2004. Ligament structure, physiology and function. *Journal of Musculoskeletal and Neuronal Interactions*, *4*(2), p. 199.

Grgic, J., Homolak, J., Mikulic, P., Botella, J. and Schoenfeld, B.J., 2018. Inducing hypertrophic effects of type I skeletal muscle fibres: A hypothetical role of time under load in resistance training aimed at muscular hypertrophy. *Medical Hypotheses*, *112*, pp. 40–42.

Herzog, W., Schappacher, G., DuVall, M., Leonard, T.R. and Herzog, J.A., 2016. Residual force enhancement following eccentric contractions: A new mechanism involving titin. *Physiology*, *31*(4), pp. 300–312.

Holzapfel, G.A., 2001. Biomechanics of soft tissue. In: Lemaitre, J. (ed.), *The handbook of materials behavior models*, Vol. 3, Boston, pp. 1049–1063.

Huxley, A.F. and Niedergerke, R., 1954. Structural changes in muscle during contraction: Interference microscopy of living muscle fibres. *Nature*, *173*(4412), pp. 971–973.

Huxley, H. and Hanson, J., 1954. Changes in the cross-striations of muscle during contraction and stretch and their structural interpretation. *Nature*, *173*(4412), pp. 973–976.

Järvinen, T.A., Järvinen, M. and Kalimo, H., 2013. Regeneration of injured skeletal muscle after the injury. *Muscles, Ligaments and Tendons Journal*, *3*(4), p. 337.

Kumka, M. and Bonar, J., 2012. Fascia: A morphological description and classification system based on a literature review. *The Journal of the Canadian Chiropractic Association*, *56*(3), p. 179.

Lang, V.A., Lundh, T. and Ortiz-Catalan, M., 2020. Mathematical models for pain: A systematic review. arXiv preprint arXiv:2006.01745.

Limbert, G., 2017. Mathematical and computational modelling of skin biophysics: A review. *Proceedings of the Royal Society A: Mathematical, Physical and Engineering Sciences*, *473*(2203), p. 20170257. http://dx.doi.org/10.1098/rspa.2017.0257

Maffulli, N., Del Buono, A., Oliva, F., Via, A.G., Frizziero, A., Barazzuol, M., Brancaccio, P., Freschi, M., Galletti, S., Lisitano, G. and Melegati, G., 2015. Muscle injuries: A brief guide to classification and management. *Translational Medicine@ UniSa*, *12*, p. 14.

Majewski-Schrage, T. and Snyder, K., 2016. The effectiveness of manual lymphatic drainage in patients with orthopaedic injuries. *Journal of Sport Rehabilitation*, *25*(1), pp. 91–97.

Mallinson, R.J. and De Souza, M.J., 2014. Current perspectives on the etiology and manifestation of the 'silent' component of the female athlete triad. *International Journal of Women's Health*, *6*, p. 451.

McCarthy, M.M. and Hannafin, J.A., 2014. The mature athlete: Aging tendon and ligament. *Sports Health*, *6*(1), pp. 41–48.

Melzack, R. and Wall, P.D., 1965. Pain mechanisms: A new theory. *Science*, Nov 19, *150*(3699), pp. 971–979.

Miake-Lye, I.M., Mak, S., Lee, J., Luger, T., Taylor, S.L., Shanman, R., Beroes-Severin, J.M. and Shekelle, P.G., 2019. Massage for pain: An evidence map. *The Journal of Alternative and Complementary Medicine*, *25*(5), pp. 475–502.

Moore Jr, J.E. and Bertram, C.D., 2018. Lymphatic system flows. *Annual Review of Fluid Mechanics*, *50*, pp. 459–482.

Mountjoy, M., Sundgot-Borgen, J., Burke, L., Carter, S., Constantini, N., Lebrun, C., Meyer, N., Sherman, R., Steffen, K., Budgett, R. and Ljungqvist, A., 2014. The IOC consensus statement: Beyond the female athlete triad—relative energy deficiency in sport (RED-S). *British Journal of Sports Medicine*, *48*(7), pp. 491–497.

Mueller-Wohlfahrt, H.W., Haensel, L., Mithoefer, K., Ekstrand, J., English, B., McNally, S., Orchard, J., van Dijk, C.N., Kerkhoffs, G.M., Schamasch, P. and Blottner, D., 2013. Terminology and classification of muscle injuries in sport: The Munich consensus statement. *British Journal of Sports Medicine*, *47*(6), pp. 342–350.

Mungal, S.U., Dube, S.P., Dhole, A., Mane, U. and Bondade, A.K., 2015. New hypothesis for mechanism of sliding filament theory of skeletal muscle contraction. *National Journal of Physiology, Pharmacy & Pharmacology*, 5(1), pp. 72–75.

Nemoto, T., Kubota, R., Murasawa, Y. and Isogai, Z., 2012. Viscoelastic properties of the human dermis and other connective tissues and its relevance to tissue aging and aging–related disease. In: De Vicente, J. (ed.), *Viscoelasticity – from theory to biological applications*, pp. 157–170. InTech. doi: 10.5772/50146. http://www.intechopencom/books/viscoelasticity-from-the ory-to- biological-applications/viscoelastic-properties-of-the-human-dermis-and-other-connect ive-tissues-and-its-relevance-to-tissue

Paddon-Jones, D., Short, K.R., Campbell, W.W., Volpi, E. and Wolfe, R.R., 2008. Role of dietary protein in the Sarcopenia of aging. *The American Journal of Clinical Nutrition*, 87(5), pp. 1562S–1566S.

Purslow, P.P., 2010. Muscle fascia and force transmission. *Journal of Bodywork and Movement Therapies*, 14(4), pp. 411–417.

Randolph, G.J., Ivanov, S., Zinselmeyer, B.H. and Scallan, J.P., 2017. The lymphatic system: Integral roles in immunity. *Annual Review of Immunology*, 35, pp. 31–52.

Roberts, T.J. and Konow, N., 2013. How tendons buffer energy dissipation by muscle. *Exercise and Sport Sciences Reviews*, 41(4), pp. 186–193. https://doi.org/10.1097/JES.0b013e3182a4e6d5

Schleip, R., Zorn, A. and Klingler, W., 2010. Biomechanical properties of fascial tissues and their role as pain generators. *Journal of Musculoskeletal Pain*, 18(4), pp. 393–395.

Shah, S. and Bhalara, A., 2012. Myofascial release. *International Journal of Health Sciences and Research*, 2(2), pp. 69–77.

Snijders, T., Nederveen, J.P., Joanisse, S., Leenders, M., Verdijk, L.B., Van Loon, L.J. and Parise, G., 2017. Muscle fibre capillarization is a critical factor in muscle fibre hypertrophy during resistance exercise training in older men. *Journal of Cachexia, Sarcopenia and Muscle*, 8(2), pp. 267–276.

Standring, S., 2008. The anatomical basis of clinical practice. *Gray's Anatomy*, 40, pp. 415–416.

Staunton, L., Zweyer, M., Swandulla, D. and Ohlendieck, K., 2012. Mass spectrometry-based proteomic analysis of middle-aged vs. aged vastus lateralis reveals increased levels of carbonic anhydrase isoform 3 in senescent human skeletal muscle. *International Journal of Molecular Medicine*, 30, 723–733.

Stecco, C. and Day, J.A., 2010. The fascial manipulation technique and its biomechanical model: a guide to the human fascial system. *International Journal of Therapeutic Massage & Bodywork*, 3(1), p. 38.

Stecco, C., Stern, R., Porzionato, A., Macchi, V., Masiero, S., Stecco, A. and De Caro, R., 2011. Hyaluronan within fascia in the etiology of myofascial pain. *Surgical and Radiologic Anatomy*, 33(10), pp. 891–896.

Stecco, C. and Schleip, R., 2016. A fascia and the fascial system. *Journal of Bodywork and Movement Therapies*, 20(1), pp. 139–140.

Stender, C.J., Rust, E., Martin, P.T., Neumann, E.E., Brown, R.J. and Lujan, T.J., 2018. Modeling the effect of collagen fibril alignment on ligament mechanical behaviour. *Biomechanics and Modeling in Mechanobiology*, 17(2), pp. 543–557.

Tresoldi, I., Oliva, F., Benvenuto, M., Fantini, M., Masuelli, L., Bei, R. and Modesti, A., 2013. Tendon's ultrastructure. *Muscles, Ligaments and Tendons Journal*, 3(1), p. 2.

Vairo, G.L., Miller, S.J., Rier, N.C.I. and Uckley, W.I., 2009. Systematic review of efficacy for manual lymphatic drainage techniques in sports medicine and rehabilitation: An evidence-based practice approach. *Journal of Manual & Manipulative Therapy*, 17(3), pp. 80E–89E.

Weinreb, J.H., Sheth, C., Apostolakos, J., McCarthy, M.B., Barden, B., Cote, M.P. and Mazzocca, A.D., 2014. Tendon structure, disease, and imaging. *Muscles, Ligaments and Tendons Journal*, 4(1), p. 66.

Wilke, J., Hespanhol, L. and Behrens, M., 2019. Is it all about the Fascia? A systematic review and meta-analysis of the prevalence of extramuscular connective tissue lesions in muscle strain injury. *Orthopaedic Journal of Sports Medicine*, 7(12), p. 2325967119888500.

Wilke, J., Macchi, V., De Caro, R. and Stecco, C., 2019. Fascia thickness, aging and flexibility: Is there an association? *Journal of Anatomy*, *234*(1), pp. 43–49.

Wisdom, K.M., Delp, S.L. and Kuhl, E., 2015. Use it or lose it: Multiscale skeletal muscle adaptation to mechanical stimuli. *Biomechanics and Modeling in Mechanobiology*, *14*(2), pp. 195–215.01023620000

3 Client Information, Assessment, Treatment Planning

Subjective, Objective, Assessment and Plan Notes

Subjective, Objective, Assessment and Plan (SOAP) note taking was devised by Harry Weed over 50 years ago and is still a widely used method of documentation for sports massage therapists and other allied professionals. However, there is minimal evidence supporting the use of subjective or objective findings as a method to identify athletes at increased risk of injury (Garrison et al., 2015). In agreement, Gossman et al. (2020) suggested that a weakness of the SOAP note is its inability to document changes over time, and rearranging the order to form APSO (Assessment, Plan, Subjective, Objective) provides the information most relevant to ongoing care at the beginning of the note where it can be found quickly, shortening the time required for the clinician to find a colleague's assessment and plan.

In the International Olympic Committee (IOC) Consensus Statement on periodic health evaluation of elite athletes, Ljungqvist et al. (2009) stated that the benefits of regular health examinations include establishing rapport between the medical team and the athlete, reviewing medications and supplements to avoid inadvertent doping, establishing a performance baseline for the athlete in the healthy state and, in some settings, satisfying the medico-legal duties of care.

Subjective – these are the experiences and views of the athlete about their condition, i.e. how they feel, where it hurts, what makes it feel better/worse.

Objective – what you observe, i.e. measurements and recordings from special tests, range of motion, posture assessment/screening, active and passive movements, strength tests (resisted movements).

Assessment – the diagnosis or identifying the problem.

Plan – interventions, referrals, follow up appointments, athlete education.

The sports massage therapist is part of a multidisciplinary team and should always operate within their scope of practice. Therefore, if the therapist has any concerns about an athlete's pathology, or other medical conditions such as unexplained weight loss, persistent headaches, urinary or bowel dysfunction, respiratory dysfunction, heart arrhythmias, circulatory disorders, significant referred pain, loss of function, a mechanical joint block, non-healing skin adhesions or night-time pain (see Chapter 4, on contraindications) they should be referred to the athlete's physician.

A history of previous injury has been the most consistent risk factor for future muscular injury in multiple sports and physical activities (Arnason et al., 2004; Maffey & Emery, 2007).

DOI: 10.4324/9781003104803-3

It has been reported that up to 63% of athletes with a past history of injury are at risk for recurrent injury (Brukner et al., 2014) with excessive and rapid increases in training load likely to be responsible for a large proportion of non-contact, soft tissue injuries (Gabbett, 2016; Drew & Finch, 2016). Therefore, it is important the therapist gets a detailed, honest reflection of the athlete's training volume, injury history and recovery procedures.

The Functional Movement Screen (FMS™) is commonly used as a predictor of future injury, but recently its use has been questioned. For example, Dorrel et al.'s 2015 systematic review and meta-analysis findings do not support the predictive validity of the FMS, due to the statistical and methodological limitations in the reviewed literature. In addition, Moran et al.'s (2017) systematic review and meta-analysis (24 studies) concluded the strength of association between FMS composite scores and subsequent injury does not support its use as an injury prediction tool. Newton et al. (2017) also suggested that the FMS should not be used for risk stratification among young elite soccer players since the composite score was unrelated to injury likelihood. However, contrary to this, Garrison et al. (2015) demonstrated a predictive relationship between FMS composite scores and past history of injury with the development of future injury.

The Functional Movement Screen consists of: deep squat, hurdle step, in-line lunge, shoulder mobility, active straight-leg raise, trunk stability push-up, rotary stability.

Testing Ranges of Motion

- Active range of motion – athlete moves the joint without assistance (see Table 3.1).
- Passive range of motion – therapist moves athlete's body part.

During a passive assessment, the therapist assists the movement performed by the athlete by supporting the limb (the athlete needs to relax to enable this to happen). The therapist then feels for impaired/restricted movements caused by pain, tightness or a mechanical 'block' within the joint, indicating a joint/cartilage related structure may be causing the problem. If there is a 'soft' end feel at the limit of the range of motion, which could be as a result of swelling, there will be a yielding compression which will prevent further movement (spongy feel). It should be remembered how body proportions and muscle bulk may affect the test and how the plane and axis of movement are oriented in space.

Resisted Movement and Strength Testing

Prior to an athlete returning to full training, muscles should be able to perform with full strength and power and without pain. For example, the assessment of strength and strength (in)balance in the knee has been used as an objective marker after anterior cruciate ligament (ACL) injury, reconstruction and subsequent rehabilitation (Huang et al., 2017). However, from 413 professional footballers tested in a study by van Dyk et al. (2017), the authors concluded that the clinical value of isolated strength testing is limited, and its use in musculoskeletal screening to predict future hamstring injury is unfounded. Therefore, the therapist should not rely on one method or type of resisted movement/strength tests when rehabilitating an athlete.

In summary, where possible assessments and re-assessments are used to measure baseline start points, progression and improvements or changes in an athlete's condition or pain level. This information can be useful for strength and conditioning coaches when planning return-to-play protocols, so care should be taken to ensure measurements are as accurate as possible.

Table 3.1 Active range of motion

Neck

Flexion	Chin to chest
Extension	Raise chin up and look at ceiling
Side rotation	Turn head to the side – left, then right
Side flexion	Move ear towards shoulder – left, then right

Shoulder girdle

Depression	Lower shoulders
Elevation	Raise shoulders
Protraction	Bring shoulders forwards
Retraction	Push shoulders back
Flexion	Move arms forwards
Extension	Move arms backwards
Abduction	Move arms outwards. Turn arm outwards across chest (horizontal abduction)
Adduction	Move arms inwards. Turn arm inwards towards chest (horizontal adduction)

Elbows

Flexion	Bend elbow
Extension	Straighten elbow

Forearms

Pronation	Turn palms downwards
Supination	Turn palms upwards

Wrists

Flexion	Bend wrist; fingers move towards palmar surface of forearm
Extension	Straighten wrist; fingers move away from forearm
Radial deviation	Bend wrist sideways by moving hand towards radius
Ulnar deviation	Bend wrist by moving hand sideways towards ulna

Fingers

Flexion	Bend fingers towards palm
Extension	Straighten fingers

Trunk

Flexion	Slump forwards (from standing), bending whole spine
Extension	Return to upright position and arch back
Side rotation	Slowly twist the spine by simultaneously moving one shoulder backwards and one forwards, keeping pelvis fixed, move left then right
Side flexion	Side bend – left, then right

Hips

Flexion	Bring upper leg forwards
Extension	Move upper leg backwards
Abduction	Move leg to the side and away from the body
Adduction	Move leg inwards towards the body
Internal rotation	Turn leg inwards
External rotation	Turn leg outwards

Knees

Flexion	Bend the knee
Extension	Straighten the knee

Feet

Inversion	Turn the sole of the foot inwards
Eversion	Turn the sole of the foot outwards

Toes

Flexion	Bend the toes towards the sole of the foot
Extension	Straighten the toes and bend upwards

References

Arnason, A., Sigurdsson, S.B., Gudmundsson, A., Holme, I., Engebretsen, L. and Bahr, R., 2004. Risk factors for injuries in football. *The American Journal of Sports Medicine*, 32(1_suppl), pp. 5–16.

Brukner, P., Nealon, A., Morgan, C., Burgess, D. and Dunn, A., 2014. Recurrent hamstring muscle injury: Applying the limited evidence in the professional football setting with a seven-point programme. *British Journal of Sports Medicine*, 48(11), pp. 929–938.

Dorrel, B.S., Long, T., Shaffer, S. and Myer, G.D., 2015. Evaluation of the functional movement screen as an injury prediction tool among active adult populations: A systematic review and meta-analysis. *Sports Health*, 7(6), pp. 532–537.

Drew, M.K. and Finch, C.F., 2016. The relationship between training load and injury, illness and soreness: A systematic and literature review. *Sports Medicine*, 46(6), pp. 861–883.

Gabbett, T.J., 2016. The training-injury prevention paradox: Should athletes be training smarter and harder? *British Journal of Sports Medicine*, 50(5), pp. 273–280.

Garrison, M., Westrick, R., Johnson, M.R. and Benenson, J., 2015. Association between the functional movement screen and injury development in college athletes. *International Journal of Sports Physical Therapy*, 10(1), p. 21.

Gossman, W., Lew, V. and Ghassemzadeh, S., 2020. SOAP notes. In: Podder, V., Lew, V. and Ghassemzadeh, S. (eds.) *StatPearls [Internet]*. Treasure Island, FL: StatPearls Publishing. Available from: https://www.ncbi.nlm.nih.gov/books/NBK482263/

Huang, H., Guo, J., Yang, J., Jiang, Y., Yu, Y., Müller, S., Ren, G. and Ao, Y., 2017. Isokinetic angle-specific moments and ratios characterizing hamstring and quadriceps strength in anterior cruciate ligament deficient knees. *Scientific Reports*, 7(1), pp. 1–11.

Ljungqvist, A., Jenoure, P., Engebretsen, L., Alonso, J.M., Bahr, R., Clough, A., De Bondt, G., Dvorak, J., Maloley, R., Matheson, G. and Meeuwisse, W., 2009. The International Olympic Committee (IOC) Consensus statement on periodic health evaluation of elite athletes. March 2009. *British Journal of Sports Medicine*, 43(9), pp. 631–643.

Maffey, L. and Emery, C., 2007. What are the risk factors for groin strain injury in sport? *Sports Medicine*, 37(10), pp. 881–894.

Moran, R.W., Schneiders, A.G., Mason, J. and Sullivan, S.J., 2017. Do Functional Movement Screen (FMS) composite scores predict subsequent injury? A systematic review with meta-analysis. *British Journal of Sports Medicine*, 51(23), pp. 1661–1669.

Newton, F., McCall, A., Ryan, D., Blackburne, C., aus der Fünten, K., Meyer, T., Lewin, C. and McCunn, R., 2017. Functional Movement Screen (FMS™) score does not predict injury in English Premier League youth academy football players. *Science and Medicine in Football*, 1(2), pp. 102–106.

van Dyk, N., Bahr, R., Burnett, A.F., Whiteley, R., Bakken, A., Mosler, A., Farooq, A. and Witvrouw, E., 2017. A comprehensive strength testing protocol offers no clinical value in predicting risk of hamstring injury: A prospective cohort study of 413 professional football players. *British Journal of Sports Medicine*, 51(23), pp. 1695–1702.

4   Contraindications and Cautions

Understanding Contraindications

Understanding contraindications to massage therapy can be a confusing area for therapists, so in all instances guidance should always be sought from the athlete's medical team if there are any doubts over previous or current medical conditions. For example, Yang et al. (2018) described how, following a vigorous back massage with spinal manipulation, a 38-year old male patient experienced cauda equina syndrome. Cauda equina syndrome (CES) is a neurological condition caused by compression of the cauda equina, most commonly described as a combination of sensory loss of the saddle area, motor deficit and/or loss of reflexes of the lower limbs, micturition dysfunction, defecation complaints and/or sexual dysfunction (Korse et al., 2013; Korse et al., 2017). The patient experienced severe numbness in both lower limbs, an inability to walk due to weakness of bilateral lower limbs and incontinence of urine and faeces (which resulted in emergency surgery). Therefore, it could be argued that massage or manipulation could worsen pre-existing herniated disc pathologies. Similarly, a 54-year-old woman presenting with a 2-month history of mild back pain required surgery following a therapeutic back massage due to the rupture of a haemorrhagic spinal angiolipoma (benign tumour) (Zhang et al., 2020).

Cherkin et al. (2001) noted that minor pain or discomfort was experienced by 13% of participants during or shortly after receiving massage. Similarly, Cambron et al. (2007) found 10% of massage clients experienced some minor discomfort after a massage session, with the majority of negative symptoms starting less than 12 hours after the massage and lasting for 36 hours or less. This highlights that not only should contraindications be understood and addressed, caution should also be applied to athletes who have not received massage before as well as those who bruise easily, have lower pain thresholds or have unexplained/undiagnosed areas of pain or discomfort.

For ease of understanding, contraindications are frequently divided into 'absolute' or 'potential' contraindications.

Absolute contraindications to massage (massage should NOT be given) include:

- Over open wounds.
- Recent stroke or heart attack.
- Intoxication (drugs or alcohol).
- Following major surgery.
- In the early stages of healing.
- Over areas of acute inflammation (muscle, tendon, heart, throat etc).
- Over-sensitive skin conditions (eczema, psoriasis).

DOI: 10.4324/9781003104803-4

- Febrile conditions (fever above 110.4°F/38°C).
- Severe unexplained internal pain.
- Unexplained weight loss.
- Acute pneumonia.
- Complications during pregnancy (eclampsia, hypertension, proteinuria, oedema).
- Haemophilia.
- Unresolved kidney or respiratory disorders.
- Metastatic cancers.
- Blood infections.
- Deep vein thrombus.
- Unexplained lumps and bumps.

Relative contraindication to massage (massage may be used with caution or under a physician's guidance) include:

- Uncontrolled hyper and hypotension.
- Diabetic complications.
- Drug withdrawal.
- When a patient is unable to consent to treatment.
- Recent traumatic brain injury.
- Joint hypermobility.
- Fragile skin.
- Compromised immune conditions (HIV).

The list above is not designed to be exhaustive. If in doubt, always refer the athlete to their appropriate physician.

Treating Athletes with Special Requirements

When working with athletes who have one or a number of special treatment requirements, including those who are pregnant, under the age of consent, elderly and those with physical or mental complications, it is common for employers to require a completed (enhanced) disclosure barring service (DBS) check. Standard DBS checks show details of spent and unspent convictions, cautions, reprimands and final warnings held on police records. Enhanced DBS checks show the same information as standard checks, plus any additional information held by local police considered relevant to the role in question. At the time of writing, this costs £35 (standard), £55.60 (enhanced) and £12 for volunteers. Some employers will require a new check every 3 years with a self-declaration completed annually. For further information in the UK, contact the Disclosure and Barring Service (https://www.gov.uk/government/organisations/disclosure-and-barring-service).

It is important to collaborate with other members of the sports and exercise medical team to fully understand the athlete's medical condition and any medication or therapeutic use exemptions (TUEs) they may be taking. In addition, a good rapport with an athlete who has special requirements should make it easier to gain information regarding any potential side effects from medications, any potential contraindications to massage or any assistance they may require getting onto the treatment couch, including positioning or turning over. Athletes with physical impairments may have an altered level of sensation, poor or no muscle tone, scarring and an altered ability to maintain their body temperature. Athletes in wheelchairs may also experience high levels of overuse injuries around the shoulders, and hand blisters from pushing their chair which may require medical attention. Additionally, it is strongly recommended that the therapist check (not presume) if amputee and lower spinal cord injured athletes require any assistance when transferring from chair to treatment couch. Song et al. (2020) reported that it is apparent the overall injury rates sustained by disabled athletes (in the Winter Paralympic Games) are high and can be comparable with injury rates in able-bodied counterparts. Therefore, therapists working with athletes with disabilities at large competitions are likely to be very busy and should familiarise themselves with as many medical conditions as possible, including the wide range of classifications at para events. For example, when treating athletes with spinal cord injuries at the T6 level and above, sports massage therapists should be aware of the condition dysreflexia. This is an uninhibited sympathetic nervous system response to a variety of noxious stimuli (described below).

Signs and symptoms include:

- Hypertension: greater than 20 mmHg above baseline for both systolic and diastolic (atypical BP in a tetraplegia patient is 90–110/60–70 mmHg in supine).
- BP is commonly lower when patient is sitting due to orthostatic hypotension.
- Severe bilateral pounding headache.
- Diaphoresis or flushing above the level of the spinal cord lesion (diaphoresis can be profuse).
- Nasal congestion.
- Visual changes or disturbances.
- Bradycardia or tachycardia (bradycardia at onset, tachycardia may follow).
- Pallor or gooseflesh below the level of the spinal cord lesion.
- Respiratory distress or bronchospasms.
- Anxiety (apprehension over impending physical problems to fear of death is common).
- Metallic taste in mouth.
- Significantly elevated BP with minimal or no symptoms (silent autonomic dysreflexia).
- For further information on autonomic dysreflexia, readers are recommended the following resource: www.spinal.co.uk.

Some athletes with acquired or congenital intellectual difficulties may have a parent or guardian who is able to assist with communication and consent to treatment, details of previous injuries and illnesses, and contraindications, as well as providing support and reassurance. In some cases, those competing with sight difficulties may have a training guide or team-mate with them to offer assistance. Likewise, those with reduced hearing may have a sign language interpreter with them to assist with communication. All athletes have the legal and ethical right to choose whether they are happy to go ahead with the therapist's assessment, treatment or referral to another practitioner. The athlete must understand why and what is going to happen during the treatment process, and any potential risks or side effects that *could* occur, so they (or their chaperone) can make any appropriate decisions. If informed consent is not sought, the therapist may be breaching legal and ethical standards, and risk legal and professional consequences.

At major sporting events it is not uncommon for athletes to have to share treatment areas, so it is important their dignity is maintained at all times. In addition, consideration of equality and diversity should be adhered to, ensuring each client is treated is fairly, appropriately and with respect. In some circumstances, especially when working with high profile athletes or teams, non-disclosure agreements (NDAs) or contracts will need to be signed to ensure confidentiality.

Is Pregnancy a Contraindication to Massage?

Pregnant athletes may wish to continue receiving massage as part of their physical preparation, recovery or injury rehabilitation throughout their pregnancy. The majority of massage courses teach students that massage is contraindicated for the first 12 weeks, but there is little to no research evidence of massage causing physical harm to the unborn child or mother during pregnancy or the postnatal period (Fogarty et al., 2019). However, as almost one-third of human embryos surviving the first 4 weeks after fertilisation are lost – some two-thirds of those before a clinical pregnancy is recognised, and one-third during the time window from clinical recognition of pregnancy until the 28th week of pregnancy (Bonde et al. 2013) – it is easy to make incorrect assumptions. This point was concurred by 20 women in a study by Fogarty and colleagues (2020), who identified features of practice that made women feel psychologically safe, such as experience and expertise, autonomy, feeling listened to, the importance of the consultation and the inclusion of specific pregnancy questions at intake.

During the first trimester, expectant mothers may have feelings of nausea and vomiting (morning sickness) at which time massage would not take place. Pregnancy complications at any time during massage should be reported to the athlete's physician immediately (see list of massage contraindications).

Numerous competitive athletes and coaches (see for example Figure 4.1) have performed at the highest level whilst pregnant:

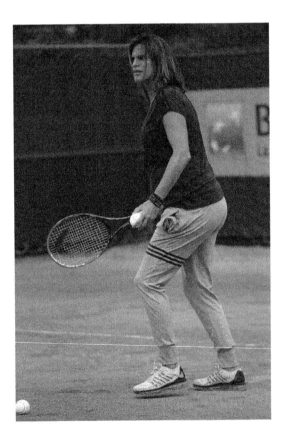

Figure 4.1 Pregnant tennis coach and two-time Grand Slam Champion Amelie Mauresmo supervises Andy Murray's practice at Roland Garros.

- Serena Williams won the Australian Open in 2017, 8 weeks pregnant.
- Kerri Walsh Jennings won a gold medal in beach volleyball at the 2012 Olympics, 6 weeks pregnant.
- Alysia Montaño ran 800m in the 2014 USA Outdoor Track and Field Championships, 34 weeks pregnant.
- Paula Radcliffe ran 14 miles a day when 5 months pregnant and ran a 10K charity run 7 months pregnant.
- Anky van Grunsven won an Olympic gold medal in dressage in Athens in 2004, 4 months pregnant.
- Martina Valcepina, short track speed skater, competed in the 2014 Sochi Games, 1 month pregnant (with twins!).
- Anna-Maria Johansson, Swedish handball player, competed in the 2012 Olympics, 3 months pregnant.
- Kristie Moore competed in the 2010 Winter Olympic Games in curling, 5 months pregnant.
- Kerstin Szymkowiak, skeleton racer, won a silver medal at the 2010 Vancouver Games, 2 months pregnant.
- Amelie Kober, snowboarder, competed in the 2010 Vancouver Games, 2 months pregnant.
- Ingrid Kristiansen won the Houston marathon (1983) 2 months pregnant.
- Sydney Leroux returned to pre-season soccer training with Orlando Pride (2018), 6 months pregnant.

Supine Hypotensive Syndrome

When massaging pregnant athletes (Figure 4.2), the therapist should be aware of supine hypotensive syndrome (also referred to as inferior vena cava compression syndrome). This is caused when the gravid uterus compresses the inferior vena cava when an expectant female is in a supine position, leading to decreased venous return centrally (Kim & Wang, 2014). As a result of this compression, blood flow returning from the extremities may be impeded drastically,

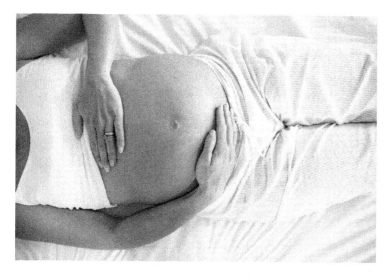

Figure 4.2 Pregnant woman holding tummy on bed.

resulting in maternal hypotension. This subsequently limits blood flow out to the placenta and may result in morbidity and mortality to the mother and foetus alike (Krywko & King, 2020). This can be avoided if the athlete lies on her left side (see Figure 4.3) during the massage or leans slightly forward in a seated position with a pillow against her chest (covered with a towel) for additional comfort (see Figures 4.4a and 4.4b). A comprehensive review of the literature (Zhao, 2014) suggested inferior vena cava (IVC) occlusion in the supine position occurs not in a minority but in the majority of women in late pregnancy. Therefore, women who are over 20 weeks should not lie in a supine position during massage.

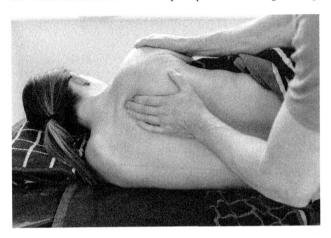

Figure 4.3 Side-lying effleurage. The right hand supports the shoulder and maintains the athlete's body position. The left hand starts with minimal pressure above the iliac crest then moves upwards towards the upper trapezius. This can be repeated 3–5 times.

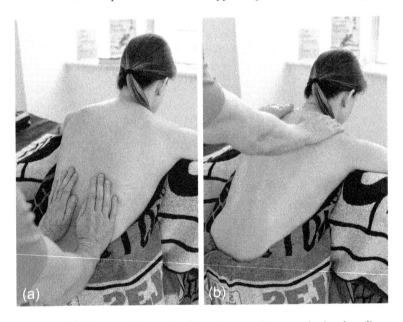

Figure 4.4 (a) Start position – the therapist starts in a crouched or kneeling position. Light pressure is used over the lower back. (b) Pressure slightly increases as both hands move upwards, parallel to the spine, towards the upper trapezius. The hands then return back to the finish position. Repeat 3–5 times.

References

Bonde, J.P.E., Jørgensen, K.T., Bonzini, M. and Palmer, K.T., 2013. Risk of miscarriage and occupational activity: A systematic review and meta-analysis regarding shift work, working hours, lifting, standing and physical workload. *Scandinavian Journal of Work, Environment & Health*, *39*(4), p. 325.

Cambron, J.A., Dexheimer, J., Coe, P. and Swenson, R., 2007. Side-effects of massage therapy: A cross-sectional study of 100 clients. *The Journal of Alternative and Complementary Medicine*, *13*(8), pp. 793–796.

Cherkin, D.C., Eisenberg, D., Sherman, K.J., Barlow, W., Kaptchuk, T.J., Street, J. and Deyo, R.A., 2001. Randomized trial comparing traditional Chinese medical acupuncture, therapeutic massage, and self-care education for chronic low back pain. *Archives of Internal Medicine*, *161*(8), pp. 1081–1088.

Fogarty, S., McInerney, C., Stuart, C. and Hay, P., 2019. The side effects and mother or child related physical harm from massage during pregnancy and the postpartum period: An observational study. *Complementary Therapies in Medicine*, *42*, pp. 89–94.

Fogarty, S., Barnett, R. and Hay, P., 2020. Safety and Pregnancy massage: A qualitative thematic analysis. *International Journal of Therapeutic Massage & Bodywork*, *13*(1), p. 4.

Kim, D.R. and Wang, E., 2014. Prevention of supine hypotensive syndrome in pregnant women treated with transcranial magnetic stimulation. *Psychiatry Research*, *218*(1–2), pp. 247–248.

Korse, N.S., Jacobs, W.C.H., Elzevier, H.W. and Vleggeert-Lankamp, C.L.A.M., 2013. Complaints of micturition, defecation and sexual function in cauda equina syndrome due to lumbar disk herniation: A systematic review. *European Spine Journal*, *22*(5), pp. 1019–1029.

Korse, N.S., Pijpers, J.A., van Zwet, E., Elzevier, H.W. and Vleggeert-Lankamp, C.L.A., 2017. Cauda Equina Syndrome: Presentation, outcome, and predictors with focus on micturition, defecation, and sexual dysfunction. *European Spine Journal*, *26*(3), pp. 894–904.

Krywko, D.M. and King, K.C., 2020. Aortocaval compression syndrome. In: *StatPearls [Internet]*. Treasure Island, FL: StatPearls Publishing. Available from: https://www.ncbi.nlm.nih.gov/books/NBK430759/

Song, Y., Zhang, W., Zhao, L., Sun, D., Huang, Y. and Gu, Y., 2020. Sports-related injuries sustained by disabled athletes in Winter Paralympic Games: A systematic review. *Journal of Medical Imaging and Health Informatics*, *10*(5), pp. 1136–1143.

Yang, S.D., Chen, Q. and Ding, W.Y., 2018. Cauda Equina syndrome due to vigorous back massage with spinal manipulation in a patient with pre-existing lumbar disc herniation: a case report and literature review. *American Journal of Physical Medicine & Rehabilitation*, *97*(4), pp. e23–e26.

Zhang, X., Wang, J.J., Guo, Y., Dong, S., Shi, W., Wang, G., Zhang, H. and Wang, G., 2020. Sudden aggravated radicular pain caused by haemorrhagic spinal angiolipomas after back massage. *World Neurosurgery*, *134*, pp. 383–387.

Zhao, P.S., 2014. Supine hypotensive syndrome: A comprehensive review of literature. *Translational Perioperative and Pain Medicine*, *1*(2), pp. 22–26.

5   Massage Techniques

Prior to discussing massage techniques, there are a few points every therapist should remember, including:

- When possible keep your back straight and bend your knees as required.
- Use your bodyweight when applying deeper pressure.
- Always maintain contact with your client when moving around the treatment couch.
- Keep your client warm – cover body parts that are not being treated.
- Use positive and professional language at all times.
- Be aware of contraindications and cautions.
- Know when you need to refer your client on to another specialist.
- Understand potential risks from different topical lotions/oils.

Topical Agents

Prior to commencing a massage, lotion, wax, cream and 'base' oils such as grapeseed and almond oil can used for skin lubrication. For patient comfort, oils and lotions should be warmed in the hands before applying to the athlete's body. Clothes should always be protected, and any residue should be thoroughly wiped off, particularly prior to performance.

Before sports participation, especially during ambient temperatures, athletes may request a sports massage with a 'heat cream/balm' to assist with their warm-up preparation. These products, designed for topical application, will typically have a methyl salicylate (MS) concentration in the region of 3–20% (Anderson et al., 2017) as their active ingredient (Figure 5.1).

Methyl salicylate (analgesic, anti-inflammatory and rubefacient/counterirritant properties) has a vasodilatory action upon absorption, resulting in an increased localised blood flow and consequently produces a rise in tissue temperature (its rubefacient action) (Wong & Rabie, 2008). Once absorbed, the resulting salicylate is distributed throughout the tissues and transcellular fluids, primarily through passive pH-dependent processes. It has been estimated that the plasma half-life for salicylate is 2 to 3 hours in low doses, increasing to 12 hours at usual anti-inflammatory doses (Anderson et al., 2017).

Particularly throughout the 1980s and 90s, the common pre-match aroma from the locker room was that of oil of wintergreen. However, its use dates back to Native Americans who used wintergreen leaves to brew tea for treating rheumatic problems, and chewed the leaves to treat respiratory conditions, headaches, sore throats, fevers, tooth decay and to augment lung capacity. There is a concern about the toxicity of wintergreen oil overdosage. Its oil contains a

DOI: 10.4324/9781003104803-5

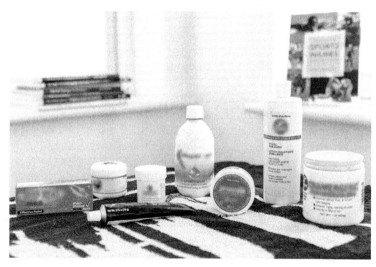

Figure 5.1 Examples of topical lotions.

high content of methyl salicylate which may be lethal if a high dosage is used (Davis, 2007). In fact, it is widely established that the ingestion of a single teaspoon (~ 5 mL) of the oil of wintergreen (98% MS), whether synthetic or natural, can be equivalent to almost 22 conventional aspirin tablets, giving rise to a potentially acute toxic dose of salicylate (Davis, 2007). One death incident has been related to excessive use of a sports cream containing high amounts of methyl salicylate. Associated Press reported (13 June 2007) a 17-year-old girl from New York died because of an overdose of methyl salicylate, caused by long term use of the sports cream 'Bengay', produced by Johnson & Johnson. The cause of death was established by health authorities in New York.

A study on the analgesic and anti-inflammatory effects of the essential oils of eucalyptus demonstrated it possesses central and peripheral analgesic effects as well as neutrophil-dependent and independent anti-inflammatory activity (Silva et al., 2003). Capsaicin and menthol are two other topically applied agents widely used for similar purposes and are known to excite and desensitise sensory nerves by acting on two members of the transient receptor potential channel superfamily (Wong & Rabie, 2008).

Hongratanaworakit (2010) recruited 40 healthy volunteers to an experimental study where jasmine oil was applied topically to the skin of the abdomen of each subject. Compared with a placebo, jasmine oil caused significant increases in breathing rate, blood oxygen saturation, and systolic and diastolic blood pressure, which indicated an increase in autonomic arousal. In addition, Kamkaen et al. (2015) noted that olfactory stimulation produces immediate changes in physiological parameters such as blood pressure, muscle tension, pupil dilation, blink magnitude, skin temperature, skin blood flow, electrodermal activity, pulse rate and brain activity.

The effects of passive rest (PR), sports massage with ozonised oil (SMOZO) and massage without ozonised oil (SM) on sports performance and psycho-physiological indices in competitive amateur cyclists, following three pre-fatiguing Wingate cycle and post-recovery ramp tests, was analysed by Paoli et al. (2013). The authors found no significant differences in cyclists' heart rate patterns in the three experimental conditions ($p > 0.05$). After SMOZO recovery, athletes showed a higher P_{max} ($p < 0.05$) and had a lower perceived fatigue visual analogue score ($p < 0.033$) in the ramp test. Blood lactate decreased more at T2 (mid-time point of treatment) and T3 (final time point of treatment) than T1 (beginning of treatment) compared to SM and PR conditions. Therefore, massaging using ozonised oil may provide some additional benefit.

Some sports, for example archery and shooting, require the athlete to be as relaxed and as focused as possible, so using some essential oils to promote this could be beneficial to performance. One oil in particular, peppermint, has been shown (Kligler & Chaudary, 2007) to be effective for relaxing and soothing muscle in the treatment of tension and headaches, and may have an action on vascular tissue; however, it could cause significant adverse effects at high dosages. Therefore, it is recommended that prior to using any essential 'aromatherapy' oil, all contraindications and precautions should be fully understood.

Cannabidiol (CBD) oil has risen in popularity over the last few years, with many therapists using it with other carrier oils (sweet almond, coconut, grapeseed, vitamin E, jojoba, calendula, chamomile, lavender, rosemary, bergamot) in various combinations. However, CBD still remains controversial, with strict restrictions in place with regard to CBD oil's tetrahydrocannabinol (THC) content. In order for CBD oil to be legal in the UK, it must contain no more than 0.2% THC, which must not be easily separated from it.

Derived from the hemp plant, cannabidiol (CBD) demonstrates anti-inflammatory and immune-modulating properties and has demonstrated to cross the blood-brain barrier and exert antioxidant, antimicrobial and neuroprotective properties. This renders it valuable in the prevention and treatment of oxidative stress associated with neurological and traumatic cerebral disorders (Reillo & Levin, 2019), and when systematically administered it reduces increases in heart rate and blood pressure induced by restraint stress (Blessing et al., 2015). In addition, Palmieri et al. (2019) demonstrated that topical treatments with CBD-enriched ointment significantly improved the quality of life of patients with several skin diseases, especially those of an inflammatory background, when they were instructed to administer topical CBD-enriched ointment to lesioned skin areas twice daily for 3 months' treatment.

Despite the lack of studies on the use of CBD in the management of sports injury, some data suggest its potential utility in osteoarthritis, delayed onset muscle soreness (DOMS) and overuse injury associated with neuropathic pain and concussion (Gamelin et al., 2020). It has been reported that in elite rugby, despite warnings from clubs and national governing bodies against CBD use, > 25% of all athletes surveyed have either used or continue to use CBD. Moreover, in the older players (> 28 years old), almost 40% have or continue to use CBD, with the major reasons cited including pain relief/recovery and to improve sleep quality (Kasper et al., 2020). Overall, existing preclinical evidence strongly supports the potential of CBD as a treatment for anxiety disorders (Blessing et al., 2015) and in achieving significant improvements in pain and other disturbing sensations (in patients with peripheral neuropathy). It is well tolerated and may provide a more effective alternative compared to other current therapies (Xu et al., 2020). Since 2018, cannabidiol has been left off WADA's prohibited list for athletes; however, tetrahydrocannabinol (THC), the better-known psychoactive component of cannabis, and its derivatives are currently still on the prohibited list, so athletes have to be mindful of the quality of the product they may consume. The threshold for a positive THC test has been set by WADA to 150 ng/mL of 11-nor-9-carboxy-THC in urine (WADA, 2013).

Effleurage – Superficial and Deep Stroking

Effleurage, a gliding or stoking technique, derives from the verb *effleurer*, which means 'to stroke'. The technique, which can be applied in a longitudinal or transverse direction, has a number of benefits, including:

- Spreading the oil or lotion.
- Increasing the temperature of the tissues.
- Improving circulation by moving venous blood towards the heart.
- Relaxing the client.
- Linking techniques together; it is used to transition between techniques.
- Assessing the structures – formulating the treatment plan.

Typically, each effleurage technique is done 3–5 times over the same area without any breaks in skin contact. Stroke rates vary depending on when the technique is used; for example, in a pre-competition setting stroke rates *could* be at around 120 strokes per minute to increase temperature and arousal. When used at the beginning of a massage or to induce relaxation the stroke rate *could* drop to 30–60 strokes per minute. On the limbs generally more pressure is applied in the direction towards the heart followed by less pressure on the return movement before the sequence is repeated, as it is believed to prevent structural damage to the valves within veins, although there is no scientific evidence to substantiate that this has ever happened during a massage. When performing deep stroking effleurage, additional bodyweight, a reinforced hand (one hand on top of the other), or the fist, knuckles or forearms can be used to stretch, reduce muscular tension and potentially re-align muscle fibres. Positive effects of effleurage have been noted, including increases in skin microcirculatory flow-motion, not only locally but also beyond, affecting systemic haemo-dynamics (Rodrigues et al., 2020); increases in sleep quality (Khoshno et al., 2016); and improved mood, due to stimulation of positive hormones and the parasympathetic nervous system which is responsible for relaxation and calmness after emotions such as stress (Field et al., 2005).

Effleurage (Superficial Stroking)

After applying oil or lotion to the hands, use even pressure with the palmar surface of the hand. Starting from the lower back on either side of the spine (see Figure 5.2a), maintain contact with the skin as the hands travel up the back (Figure 5.2b), over the shoulders (see Figure 5.2c), and return back to the start position. Repeat 3–5 times.

Effleurage (Deep Stroking)

Starting on the left of the athlete, use your left hand on top of your right to give reinforcement (Figure 5.3a). Using your bodyweight, apply deeper stroking movements along the length of the upper back parallel to the vertebrae. The amount of pressure should be dictated by the athlete's requirements, pain tolerance level and desired outcome. This technique can be applied in small sections and can also be used around the medial scapula border. To apply greater pressure, the forearm or elbow can be used (Figure 5.3b) if necessary. Repeat until the muscle tissue relaxes. Change hands to work on the opposite side of the back or move to the opposite side of the treatment couch.

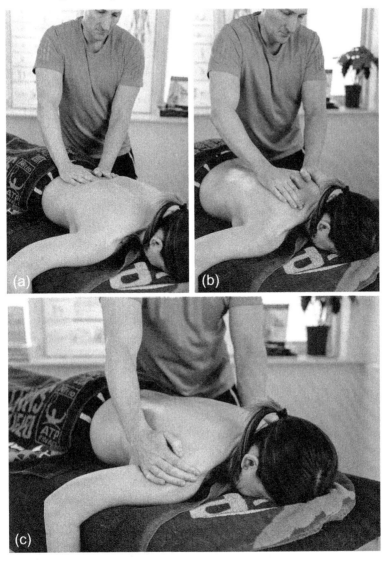

Figure 5.2 (a) Starting from the lower back either side of the spine. (b) Maintain contact with the skin as the hands travel up the back over the shoulders. (c) Return back to the start position.

Again, to apply deep stroking, standing at the head end of the treatment couch, the hands, or closed fists (if greater pressure is required) glide down towards the sacrum (Figure 5.4a). At this point the hands/closed fists glide back to the start position. Repeat 3–5 times. The technique can also be used from the sacrum working up the length of the back (Figure 5.4b).

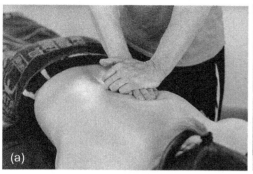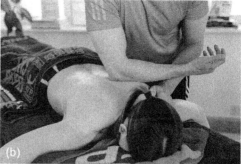

Figure 5.3 (a) Reinforced hand. (b) Using the forearm (avoid bony areas).

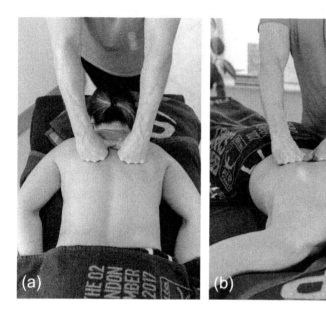

Figure 5.4 (a and b) Using closed fists

Figure-of-Eight Effleurage

Both hands start just above the sacrum (Figure 5.5a), then glide up towards the upper trapezius (Figure 5.5b). The hands go wide over the shoulder area (Figure 5.5c) and cross, completing a figure of eight motion (Figure 5.5d) Repeat 3–5 times.

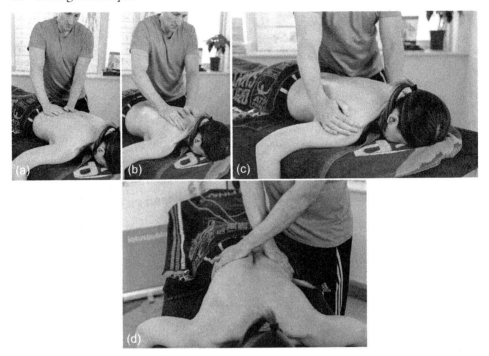

Figure 5.5 (a) Both hands start just above the sacrum. (b) Glide up towards the upper trapezius. (c) The hands go wide over the shoulder area. (d) Cross completing figure of eight motion.

Deep Stroking – Latissimus Dorsi

Starting at the head end of the couch, hold onto the athlete's right arm just under the elbow (be aware of shoulder mobility restrictions). Use your left hand (as shown in Figure 5.6a) to apply a deep stroking technique down the lateral side of the body(as far as you can comfortably reach; see Figure 5.6b), covering the latissimus area. Repeat 3–4 times.

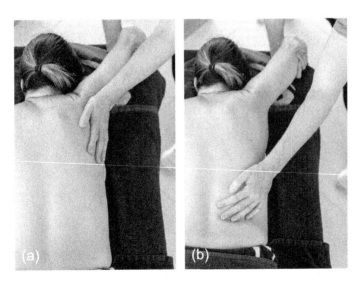

Figure 5.6 (a and b) Use your left hand to apply a deep stroking technique down covering the latissimus area.

Deep Stroking – Upper Trapezius

Using a reinforced hand for increased pressure, slowly pull the hands back towards you along the length of the upper trapezius towards the acromion process (see Figure 5.7). Repeat as necessary covering all of the upper trapezius.

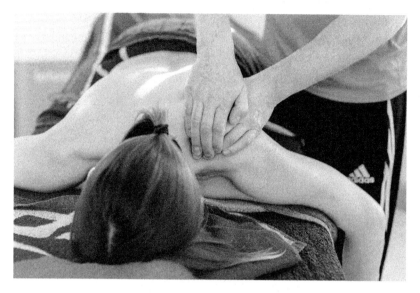

Figure 5.7 Deep stroking – upper trapezius.

Effleurage – Posterior Legs

Long flowing movements are performed to warm the tissues. The hands start from either above the knee or the Achilles tendon (in prone), moving from distal to proximal towards the ischial tuberosity (Figure 5.8). Remember to reduce the pressure when massaging behind the

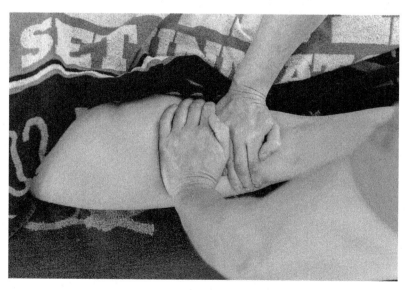

Figure 5.8 The hands start from either above the knee or the achilles tendon (in prone), from distal to proximal towards the ischial tuberosity.

knee (popliteal fossa). The hands should maintain contact with the skin at all times, and pressure can be gradually increased as more strokes are performed. The hands should glide back with minimal pressure to the start position. Repeat 3–5 times.

Deeper stroking techniques can be performed over all the hamstring muscles using a reinforced hand, fingers or thumb (Figure 5.9). Repeat 3–5 times.

Superficial effleurage to the adductors is shown in Figure 5.10. The athlete's leg should be supported by towels under the knee (if flexibility allows) or the athlete's knee can be placed on towels on the therapist's stomach. The hands sweep from distal to proximal. The left hand moves across to the left and the right hand moves across to the right, staying slightly lower than the left hand. Good towel management is required at all times. This technique is repeated 3–5 times.

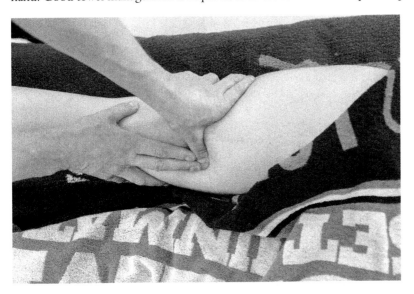

Figure 5.9 Deeper stroking techniques can be performed over all the hamstring muscles using a reinforced hand, fingers or thumb.

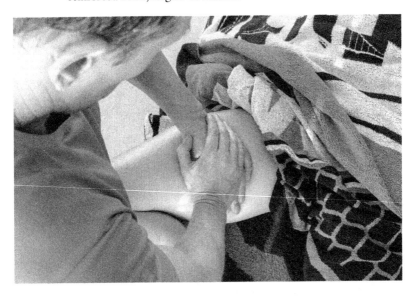

Figure 5.10 Superficial effleurage to the adductors.

Effleurage (deep stroking) is shown in Figure 5.11. The fingers add pressure to the thumb to apply deeper work through the adductors from distal to proximal in small sections at a time. This can be repeated as necessary.

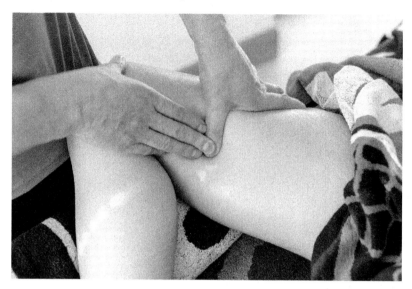

Figure 5.11 Effleurage (deep stroking).

Arms – Superficial Stroking

One hand holds the athlete's wrist whilst the other moves along the flexor side of the forearm, as shown in Figure 5.12. To work on the extensor side, change hands and pronate the athlete's

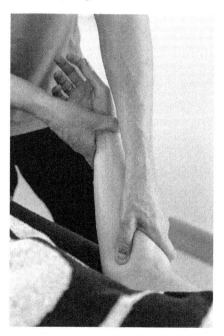

Figure 5.12 One hand holds the athlete's wrist whilst the other moves along the flexor side of the forearm.

wrist. Repeat 3–5 times on each side of the forearm. Deeper work using circular frictions can then be performed.

Effleurage (Deep Stroking) – Pectorals

After superficial effleurage to the pectoral area, place one hand on top of the other (Figure 5.13). Locate the pectoral muscle between the rib spaces and pull the muscle back towards the shoulder area, covering as much of the muscle tissue as possible. Repeat as necessary.

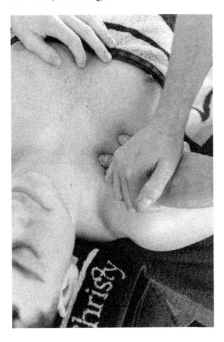

Figure 5.13 After superficial effleurage to the pectoral area, place one hand on top of the other.

Petrissage – Picking Up and Squeezing, Wringing, Skin Rolling

Petrissage, from the French word *pétrir* (to knead), is a vigorous stroke which compresses and releases the soft tissue by picking up and squeezing the muscle and overlying tissues. It is aimed at stretching muscle fibres, increasing mobility between the tissue interfaces, aiding venous and lymph return, relaxing muscle, helping with the removal of waste products (Paine, 2000) and drawing new blood and oxygen into the tissues (Zhong et al., 2019). One or both hands can be used to squeeze, lift and compress the muscle in a rhythmical manner, with the amount of pressure dependent on the area being treated and the athlete's tolerance. Petrissage follows effleurage techniques, with stroke rates adjusted for pre- or post-competition requirements. Research has indicated that petrissage may improve cycle ergometer pedalling performance, aiding improved recovery from muscle stiffness and experienced lower-limb fatigue (Ogai et al., 2008).

Petrissage – Back

When kneading (picking up and squeezing), the underlying tissue is lifted, squeezed and released, using each hand alternately in a circular motion to raise tissue temperature and increase local circulation. Stroke rates can be increased for pre-competition massage or be slowed down during recovery sessions. As with all petrissage techniques, it is important not to pinch or trap the tissue between the hands or thumbs.

The therapist's feet move when transitioning from effleurage to petrissage by moving to face the side of the massage couch, with the knees kept slightly bent. Use both hands in a rhythmical 'wave like' motion (as if baking bread) in a large circular motion from the shoulder/upper back area to the lower back, then move to the side of the lower back nearest to you, followed by the upper back/shoulder area again. Repeat as necessary. This technique is shown in Figures 5.14a and 5.14b.

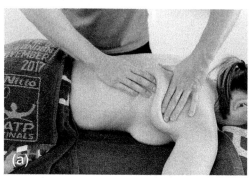 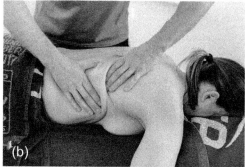

Figure 5.14 (a and b) The therapist's feet move when transitioning from effleurage to petrissage by moving to face the massage couch, with the knees kept slightly bent.

Petrissage – Upper Trapezius

As shown in Figure 5.15, the hands continually work with the thumbs grasping and releasing the bulk of the muscle. To work the opposite trapezius it may be possible to reach across the athlete, or move around to the other side of the treatment couch.

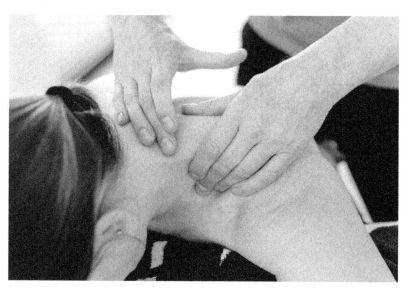

Figure 5.15 The hands continually work with the thumbs grasping and releasing the bulk of the muscle.

Petrissage – Legs

When applying large circular frictions over the length of the hamstrings (from distal to proximal) the thumb of the left hand is uppermost and sweeps away to the left, while the thumb on the right hand sweeps around, slightly down, and across to the right (see Figure 5.16). At the top of the limb the hand drags gently down the leg and the motion is repeated. This technique can also be applied using the heel of the hand rather than the thumbs with various amounts of pressure, depending on the desired outcome.

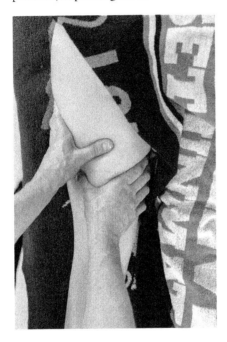

Figure 5.16 When applying large circular frictions over the length of the hamstrings (from distal to proximal) the thumb of the left hand is uppermost and sweeps away to the left, the thumb on the right hand sweeps around, slightly down, and across to the right.

As shown in Figures 5.17a and 5.17b, the tissue is manipulated in a 'wave-like' motion until all the posterior leg has been covered, using the same technique previously described alongside

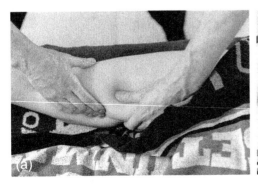 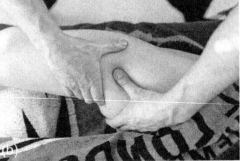

Figure 5.17 (a and b) The tissue is manipulated in a 'wave-like' motion until all the posterior leg has been covered, using the same technique previously described in Figures 5.14a and 5.14b.

Figures 5.14a and 5.14b. The therapist lets their own body sway from side to side during the technique, whilst keeping the knees slightly bent at all times. This technique can be used on the anterior thigh/adductor area.

Wringing

Both hands pull and push the muscle tissue before releasing it and continuing the motion along the length of the muscle. By lifting and squeezing, wringing is used to help improve the condition of muscles by aiding venous return, removing waste products and increasing tissue elasticity.

Skin Rolling

The skin is rolled between the thumbs and fingers of both hands, usually on larger areas of the body, for example the back. The therapist uses their thumbs, adducts and presses (rolls) the thumbs forward in order to 'bunch' up the skin, then releases and continues this sequence until the area has been covered sufficiently to stretch the subcutaneous fascia.

Tapotement – Hacking, Striking, Pounding, Slapping

Tapotement, derived from the French word *tapoter* (to tap or give a light blow), involves brisk percussions used in a rapid, alternating and rhythmical fashion. This is done by either chopping the area with the sides (ulnar borders) of the hands or striking with cupped, loosely fisted hands, palms, or fingers. Avoid bony areas, the abdominal region, kidneys and other sensitive areas. This technique can be applied directly onto the skin, through towels or over clothes, and is used to stimulate nerve endings, increase circulation and leave the athlete physically and mentally invigorated.

- Hacking – performed using the ulnar side (little finger side) of the hand in alternating blows with the wrists and fingers kept loose. See Figure 5.18.

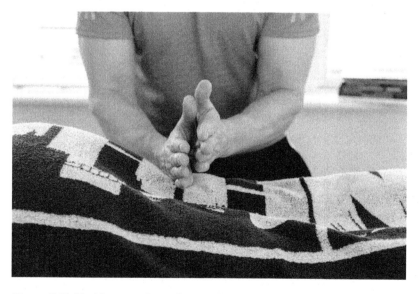

Figure 5.18 Hacking – performed using the ulnar side (little finger side) of the hand in alternating blows with the wrists and fingers kept loose.

- Cupping – performed with the palmar side of the hand in a concave position. This technique is frequently used over the posterior rib cage in chronic lung conditions, for example, cystic fibrosis, to loosen mucus in the air passages. See Figure 5.19.

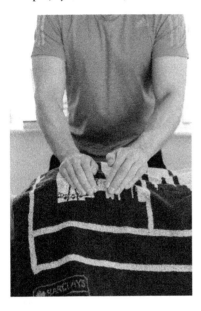

Figure 5.19 Cupping – performed with the palmar side of the hand in a concave position.

- Pounding – loose fists rotate over each other (similar to using a boxing speed ball). See Figure 5.20.

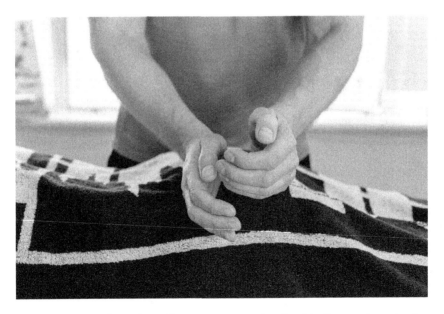

Figure 5.20 Pounding – loose fists rotate over each other (similar to using a boxing speed ball).

- Slapping – performed with the palmar side of the hand using more finger surface than palm.
- Tapping – performed using the fingertips.

Vibrations

Static vibrations involve using the therapist's whole hand or part of the hand to apply continuous contact with the athlete's body, without sliding over the skin. Running vibrations are very similar, but there is a slight glide over the skin where the tissues are pressed and released in an up and down movement. Hand-held deep oscillation massage devices have also been used as a way of self-administering vibration massage. A study by Kraft et al. (2013) of patients with moderate to severe grades of fibromyalgia syndrome (FMS) showed vibration massage to be safe, well tolerated and highly accepted.

Frictions

Friction massage (pioneered by Cyriax) deliberately causes tissue damage, hyperaemia and mild inflammation and is used to increase circulation and release areas that are tight, particularly around joints, muscles, fascia or tendons where there are chronic adhesions. Frictions can be applied transversely across soft tissue structures, in a circular movement, or with deep or superficial pressure, depending on the desired outcome; these techniques are shown in Figures 5.21, 5.22 and 5.23 Deep friction massage is given in a transverse direction to the fibre orientation in order to mobilise the fibres.

When using transverse frictions on an athlete, use a reinforced thumb or index finger (see Figure 5.21) making firm contact on the skin without lotion, at a rate of approximately

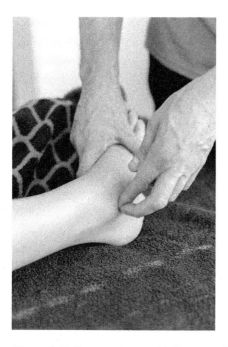

Figure 5.21 Deep transverse friction over the lateral ankle ligaments.

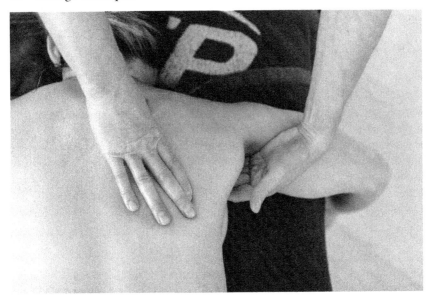

Figure 5.22 Deep circular frictions (not to be confused with deep transverse frictions) can be used on the serratus anterior. This technique can also be used with athletes in a supine or a side lying position. In prone, the right hand pushes the scapula across (laterally) and the fingers of the left hand complete small circular frictions in an upward direction.

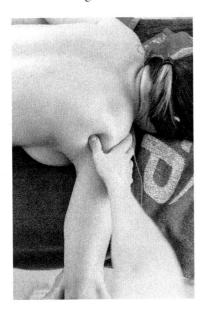

Figure 5.23 Small circular frictions over the infraspinatus and teres minor area.

2–3 frictions per second for 10 minutes every third day (for chronic injuries). In an acute phase, transverse friction massage is applied until analgesia, and from that point (once target tissue is reached) six sweeps (frictions) more (Pitsillides & Stasinopoulos, 2019). The pressure should be deep enough to move the tissue back and forth firmly and should be tolerable to the athlete. After a few minutes they should get an analgesic effect, at which time the therapist is able to increase the pressure to affect deeper tissue. When targeting the deeper layers of the tissue, the thumbs, fingertips, knuckles, palms or elbows can be used in larger deep circular movements to manipulate muscular areas. The effects of deep transverse friction massage (DTFM) were compared to both static stretching and dynamic stretching (Fakhro et al., 2020) on hamstring extensibility, agility (T-drill) and strength (1 rep max) in 103 football players. The participants received the intervention sessions three times per week for a total of 12 sessions over a 4-week period. DTFM showed improvements but did not outweigh the effects on footballers' performance when compared to static and dynamic techniques.

Soft Tissue Release/Active Release Therapy (ART)®

Active Release Therapy, also known as Active Release Technique, is a soft tissue system/movement-based technique developed and patented by P. Michael Leahy (Trivedi et al., 2014). During ART, deep digital tension is applied to the affected structure as it is moved from a shortened to a lengthened position. The treatment goal is to improve or restore soft tissue dysfunction by reducing tissue stiffness, fibrosis or adhesions.

There are three types of soft tissue/active release:

- Passive – the therapist instigates movement.
- Active – the client instigates movement whilst the therapist assists.
- Weight-bearing – the client instigates movement while the therapist assists.

Ensuring the muscle is in a neutral position, the therapist applies pressure to the muscle to form a temporary false attachment point, or lock (starting proximally on or near the origin). The therapist brings the muscle into a pain-free stretch in order to lengthen, untangle and rearrange specific muscle fibres. During active treatments the therapist may apply direct pressure to the affected area and instruct the athlete to perform a movement.

In a study of 24 patients with chronic neck pain, Kim et al. (2015) compared ART, joint mobilisations (JM), and no treatment using visual analogue scale (VAS) scores, pressure pain threshold (PPT) and range of motion (ROM). The study revealed that ART and JM both positively affected the VAS score, PPT and ROM, and the two methods demonstrated few significant differences in their effects. However, ART demonstrated a trend toward greater effectiveness for patients with neck pain. In another study, a single session of the Active Release Technique improved hamstring flexibility and range of motion in the popliteal angle ($p < 0.001$) and in a sit and reach flexibility test ($p < 0.001$) (Kage & Ratnam, 2014). Furthermore, positive results were also demonstrated in a study of 60 patients of mixed gender (age = 20–50): two groups (one undergoing myofascial release [MFR] and the other undergoing active release) noted VAS score improvements on the seventh day following the interventions. The group receiving ART showed more significant improvements in neck range of motion ($p < 0.001$), neck disability index ($p < 0.0001$) and VAS score ($p < 0.0001$) when compared to the group which received MFR (Mishra et al., 2018).

The effectiveness of back pain and/or leg pain treatment using active soft tissue release alone or in combination with a trigger point block was examined (Kameda & Tanimae, 2019) in a study of 115 patients. The gluteus medius was the major myofascial trigger point in all groups. The authors concluded that manual therapy with active soft tissue release and a trigger point block constitutes an effective treatment combination for low back pain and leg pain, but that prolonged treatment is required in chronic cases. Finally, Sadria et al. (2017) concluded that both ART and muscle energy technique (MET) equally reduced symptoms of latent trigger points (LTrPs; see the discussion of myofascial trigger points later in the chapter) in the upper trapezius in two groups by increasing active range of cervical lateral flexion ($p < 0.001$), decreasing pain intensity on VAS ($p < 0.05$) and decreasing thickness of the upper trapezius muscle ($p < 0.01$).

Before firm conclusions can be drawn on the effectiveness of using soft tissue therapy or active release techniques further well designed and controlled studies are needed, as currently a number of articles are either case studies, pilot studies, were not randomised, or failed to include a control group.

Examples of Soft Tissue Release Techniques

Pectoralis Major

Place the fist or heel of the hand on the pectoralis muscle (lock) then slowly take the athlete's arm away from their body (abduction). As the fibres of the pectoralis major vary in direction the therapist needs to change the angles of abduction (any shoulder discomfort and the athlete's range of motion will dictate the amount of range possible). Pain-free external rotation movements can also be added with the lock in place. Repeat 3–5 times as necessary. The technique is shown in Figures 5.24a and 5.24b.

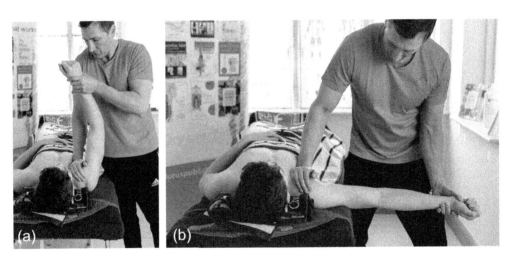

Figure 5.24 (a) Start. (b) Finish.

Bicep Brachii

Once the lock has been applied to the biceps (with the fingers, loose fist or open hand) slowly straighten the arm (Figures 5.25a and 5.25b). Repeat as necessary.

Forearm Extensors

Apply the lock with the wrist and fingers in an extended position (Figure 5.26a). Ask the athlete to slowly flex the wrist and fingers (Figure 5.26b). Vary the position of the lock and repeat as necessary.

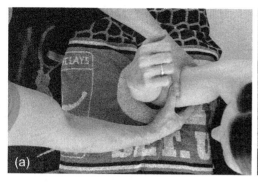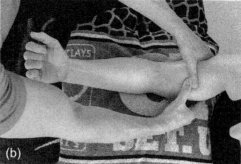

Figure 5.25 (a) Start. (b) Finish.

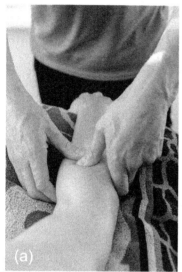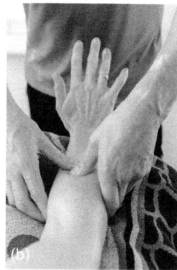

Figure 5.26 (a) Start. (b) Finish.

Positional Release Therapy/Strain-Counterstrain Technique

Positional release therapy (PRT) is described by Amini et al. (2017) as 'an indirect and passive manual technique which uses tender points and comfort position to relieve musculoskeletal pain and related dysfunctions'. It is a passive technique that places body part in a position of ease or greatest comfort, relieving pain. This position of minimal discomfort is usually the position in which muscle is at its shortest length and held for 90 seconds, following this the joint is slowly and passively returned to its neutral position. This prolonged shortening causes shortening of both intrafusal and extrafusal fibers, which in turn results in significant increase in range of motion and decrease in pain (Kannabiran 2015).

There are three main techniques used in positional release, usually used in combination: strain-counterstrain (SCS), facilitated positional release (FPR) and technical and functional technique (TF).

SCS has been described as an indirect technique that uses passive body positioning of spastic muscles and dysfunctional joints toward positions of comfort that compress or shorten the malfunctioning structure, hence relaxing the aberrant reflexes and alleviating pain (Zein-Hammoud & Standley, 2015). However, the scientific evidence behind positional release/strain-counterstrain is still in its infancy and has indicated mixed results. For example, when PRT was compared with manual passive muscle shortening (MPMS) using a double-blind randomised controlled trial on 30 female university students, both MPMS and PRT were effective techniques in immediate pain relief of upper-trapezius myofascial tripper points (MTrPs), with no significant differences between the groups ($p > 0.05$) (Amini et al., 2017). Additionally, there were no differences between the SCS, sham SCS and dry needling (DN) groups in any of the outcome measures for active myofascial trigger points in the upper trapezius in a study by Segura-Orti et al. (2016). Dry needling relieved pain after fewer sessions than SCS and sham SCS, and thus may be a more efficient technique. Also, when comparing the effectiveness of muscle energy technique, ischaemic compression and SCS with conventional therapy on upper trapezius trigger points in 45 patients with mechanical neck pain, Kumar et al. (2015) concluded that muscle energy technique is superior to ischaemic compression and SCS techniques ($p < 0.05$).

In research comparing the efficacy of ART with ultrasound, SCS, and ultrasound only on latent trigger points in the upper trapezius, Bookwala et al. (2015) demonstrated that all three treatments were deemed effective in 60 subjects, with ART and SCS more effective than the ultrasound-only treatment. Another study of 99 subjects, assessing the short-term effects on mandibular dynamics (in terms of mouth opening [MO] and bite force [BF]) compared to a placebo, Gerez et al. (2019) suggested that muscular inhibition methods by the application of SCS could be used in the treatment of MTrPs of the masseter, temporalis and internal pterygoid muscles. The authors concluded that SCS methods offer some advantages in comparison with ischemic compression techniques. The latter requires the muscle to be in a pre-tensioned (or stretched) position, whereas SCS methods are usually applied to relaxed muscles. Ischemic compression is usually painful whereas SCS does not normally cause pain, so SCS methods should be applied to increase the muscular force of the mandibular closure muscles.

Meanwhile, five randomised control trials were included in a systematic review and meta-analysis (Wong et al. 2014) to determine the pooled effect of SCS on trigger point palpation pain, compared to a control condition. The authors found low-quality evidence suggesting SCS may reduce trigger point palpation pain. Therefore, using positional release techniques/SCS *may* have a place in the therapist's treatment toolkit, and could be particularly useful for athletes who find direct sustained ischemic pressure too uncomfortable. However, low-quality evidence and mixed results indicate that these techniques are unlikely to offer greater benefits than any other form of treatment.

Myofascial Release

Prior to myofascial techniques being discussed, it is important to understand the importance of the autonomic and central nervous systems during this method of treatment. Confusingly, foam rolling (discussed in Chapter 11) is frequently reported as self-myofascial release; therefore, in this section only, the effects of foam rolling on the nervous system have also been considered.

Autonomic Nervous System

Rolling-induced mechanisms to increase range of motion or reduce pain include the activation of cutaneous and fascial mechanoreceptors and interstitial type III and IV afferents that modulate sympathetic/parasympathetic activation, as well as the activation of global pain modulatory systems and reflex-induced reductions in muscle and myofascial tone (Behm and Wilke, 2019). Myofascial release proponents believe stimulating these receptors reduces sympathetic tone, increases gamma motor neuron activity and reduces tissue viscosity (Schleip, 2003a) and promotes the relaxation of intra-fascial smooth muscle cells (Schleip, 2003b). It has also been reported that the autonomic nervous system promotes vasodilation and local fluid dynamics which alter the viscosity of fascia by changing the ground substance to a more gel-like state (Schleip, 2003b). This reduces friction between muscle fibres and creates ease of motion (Shah & Bhalara, 2012).

Central Nervous System

The central nervous system's role in MFR is more clearly understood than that of the autonomic nervous system. When the mechanoreceptors are stimulated, activation of both the autonomic nervous system and the central nervous systems occur simultaneously. The central nervous system's response to localised pressure is well known to include changing the tonus in some related striated muscle fibres (Schleip, 2003b). This leads to the proposed 'release' felt through the application of MFR.

The forearms are used (with additional bodyweight) to slowly 'spread' the tissues (Figure 5.27a). The forearms slowly rotate and spread the tissue, using a supinated to pronated position (Figure 5.27b). The direction of tension should also be changed by following the 'feel' of muscle restrictions.

The same technique can also be performed using the hands, by moving from the iliac crest across the back and finishing on the opposite upper thoracic area (Figure 5.28). Repeat as necessary.

From a therapeutic standpoint, myofascial release (MFR) is a form of manual therapy that involves the application of a low load, long-duration stretch to the myofascial chain (as shown in Figures 5.27a and 5.27b) with the aim of restoring optimal length, decreasing pain and improving function, with techniques being held for 90–120 seconds (Sullivan et al., 2013).

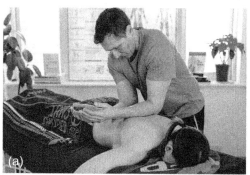 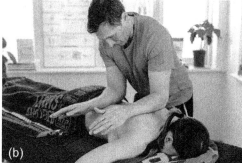

Figure 5.27 (a) Start position. (b) Finish position.

The myofascia must be 'engaged' with just the right force and at just the right angle. This is a process of 'taking up the slack' to the point that a very slight resistance is felt. Once the tissues are engaged, a manual force (usually traction) is applied in such a way that one feels the myofascia release (Kidd et al., 2009).

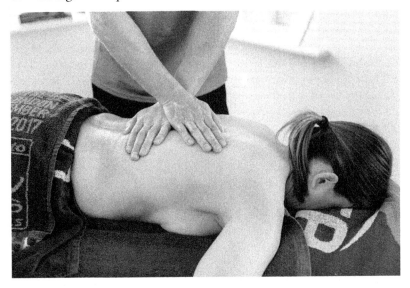

Figure 5.28 The same technique can also be performed using the hands, by moving from the iliac crest across the back, and finishing on the opposite upper thoracic area.

Laimi et al.'s 2018 systematic review of eight relevant studies ($n = 457$) concluded, due to poor effect size and risk of bias, that the current evidence on myofascial release therapy is not sufficient to warrant using the treatment for chronic musculoskeletal conditions. In another systematic review, by Ajimsha et al. (2015), the authors also suggested that the literature regarding the effectiveness of MFR was mixed in both quality and results. However, they did conclude that MFR is emerging as a strategy with a solid evidence base and tremendous potential. On a positive note, the effects of four sessions of MFR treatments, each lasting 40 minutes, on patients with non-specific low back pain was studied by Arguisuelas et al. (2017). In this study, results indicated MFR produced a significant improvement in both pain and disability.

Trivedi et al. (2016) proposed that 4 weeks of MET and MFR treatment was effective in reducing pain ($p < 0.05$) and improving the range of motion ($p < 0.05$) in mouth opening in patients suffering from temporomandibular dysfunction (TMD). However, the MET group was superior compared to MFR and a control group, with the authors believing this may be because MET stimulates muscle spindles and Golgi tendon organs, reducing excessive activity.

Myofascial release techniques are frequently used to elongate the tissues (fascia) through the facial slings; however, as Chaudhry et al. (2008) indicated, the problem of reversibility arises. In colloidal substances, the thixotropic softening effect lasts only as long as the pressure or heat is applied; after the application of heat or force, the substance returns to its state of previous rigidity within minutes. This means any potential benefits from using myofascial techniques may be short-lived. Studies have shown that in order to achieve a permanent elongation of collagen fibres one needs to apply an extremely forceful stretch of 3–8% fibre elongation, which would result in tissue tearing along with inflammation and other side effects that are usually seen as undesirable in a myofascial session (Schleip, 2003a). Alternatively, therapeutic sessions would need to take longer than an hour (which could be taken at several intervals) with softer 1–1.5% fibre elongation to achieve permanent deformation without tearing and inflammation (Thelkeld, 1992). Interestingly, Zein-Hammound and Standley (2015) found lower magnitude (3–6%) and longer duration (≥ 5 minutes) of MFR was shown to improve wound healing in vitro. This mechanism could be attributed to changes in the extracellular matrix (e.g.

collagen synthesis, secretion and architecture) and gene activation that might result from MFR applied for longer than 2 minutes.

From a treatment perspective, Chaudhry et al. (2014) made an important point. Skin experiences more compression and shear – about 1.5 times as much as the fascia – and the adipose tissue experiences about 2.5 to 3.5 times the deformation of the fascia when subjected to a specified force. However, because these tissues are incompressible, they must deform differently in the lateral direction, but in reverse, to maintain a constant volume. This information is important to consider, as it implies that the tissue impact in the lateral direction is quite different from that in the longitudinal direction and perpendicular to the skin. Therefore, the direction and pressure of the technique used by therapists may be important in achieving the desired clinical outcome.

The evidence behind the use of myofascial techniques generally has not been positive. However, much depends on the innate talent and experience of the therapist. Even if all diagnostic variables could be controlled, any difference in outcome would have to be ascribed to the manual therapist using a particular technique, rather than to the technique itself (Kidd, 2009).

Myofascial Trigger Points

Myofascial trigger points are foci of muscles that have intense sensitivity and irritability, are located predominantly near the motor end plates, and have palpable tensile band characteristics mediated by the local response of reflex muscle contraction upon palpation of muscle fibres (Wada et al., 2020). MTrP therapy is a localised form of ischemic compression (IC) applied to adhesions or 'knots' in the muscle known as 'trigger points,' which become taut and appear to adhere themselves to surrounding tissue. A prevailing hypothesis regarding the pathogenesis of MTrPs states that muscle injury or overload results in excessive acetylcholine release from motor end plates (Shokri et al., 2015). Sarcomere length is reduced, width is increased and the sustained contractions of muscle sarcomeres compress local blood supply, restricting the energy needs of the local region (Vijayakumar et al., 2019). The purpose of applying ischemic compression is to increase local blood flow upon release, which is believed to facilitate the removal of waste products, supply oxygen and promote healing of the tissue (Montañez-Aguilera et al., 2010). This deep pressure could offer effective stretching and mobilisation of the taut bands (Khan et al., 2020) which in patients with myofascial pain could be 50% greater than that of the surrounding tissue (Chen et al., 2007).

A trigger point is described as active or latent depending on its reproduction of clinical symptoms rather than the presence of spontaneous pain (Fernández-de-las-Peñas & Dommerholt, 2018). Active trigger points tend to hurt spontaneously during activity as well as at rest (Morihisa et al., 2016; Onik et al., 2020). They are usually formed by a chronic or acute overload of the muscles and are observed mostly among younger athletes. By contrast, latent trigger point pain is reproducible by palpation (Morihisa et al., 2016; Onik et al., 2020). For example, these trigger points only start hurting if there is a provoking event, such as injury, infection or another type of stressor, and are usually observed among non-athletic and older populations.

Fifty-eight male students participated in a single-blind randomised clinical trial comparing the short-term effect of Kinesio-taping versus friction massage on latent trigger points in the upper trapezius muscle (Mohamadi et al., 2017). The authors recorded pressure pain threshold with a pressure algometer, and grip strength was recorded with a Colin dynamometer. Results indicated that three sessions of either of the two interventions did not improve latent trigger points; in fact, the decrease in pressure pain threshold in both groups may indicate that these interventions not only failed to ameliorate latent trigger points but may have stimulated these points or attracted participants' attention to their pain.

Moraska et al. (2017) investigated subjects ($n = 62$) with episodic or chronic tension-type headaches. The subjects were randomised to receive 12 twice-weekly 45-minute massages, sham ultrasound sessions or a wait-list control. Massage focused on trigger point release (ischemic compression) of MTrPs in the bilateral upper trapezius and suboccipital muscles. Pressure pain threshold was measured at MTrPs with a pressure algometer pre, and post, the first and final (12th) treatments. The authors concluded that both single and multiple massage applications increased PPT at MTrPs. In agreement, a systematic review by Peta and Cardoso (2020) (from eight randomised articles) also suggested ischemic compression plays a fundamental role in the treatment of the trigger point presented in the upper trapezius. Conversely, Mohamadyari et al. (2018) examined the effects of two methods of sports massage and cold stretch on pressure pain threshold in passive trigger points in the shoulder girdle muscles of 32 national female volleyball players. In this study, both interventions had no significant effect on the pressure pain threshold in passive trigger points. Additionally, a study by Benito-de-Pedro et al. (2020) revealed that there were no differences between ischemic compression and deep dry needling ($p > 0.05$) for ankle dorsiflexion range of motion in the calf muscle (tricep surae) in 34 triathletes.

Patients with acute lower back pain received superficial effleurage massage three times a week for two weeks, with or without compression at MTrPs. The patients completed visual analogue scales, pressure pain threshold at trigger points, a Roland-Morris questionnaire (RMQ), and a range of motion test. The authors concluded that static and dynamic VAS scores, PPT and ROM were significantly improved in the MTrP group compared with those in the non-MTrP and effleurage groups (Takamoto et al., 2015). Further positive results were documented in a systematic review by Cagnie et al. (2015). Pub Med and Web of Science databases were searched to compare ischemic compression and dry needling on MTrPs in the upper trapezius muscle in patients with neck pain. From the authors' review, ischemic compression and dry needling can both be recommended in the treatment of neck pain. However, the authors did state that additional research with high-quality study designs are required to develop conclusive evidence. Furthermore, combination therapies (muscle energy technique plus ischemic compression therapy [ICT]) showed immediate and short-term (2-week follow-up) improvements in neck pain and muscle tenderness in male patients with upper trapezius active MTrPs in a study by Alghadir et al. (2020).

Aside from the hypothesis of excessive acetylcholine release from motor end plate noise on the physiological mechanism underlying myofascial trigger points, the causes of a palpable 'release' following treatment have not been fully explained. However, the research does indicate that effleurage, stretching (MET), ischemic compression and dry needling do provide some relief from trigger point discomfort, although clearly further research is warranted, with Li et al. (2020) highlighting a lack of transparency in the reporting of MTrP diagnostic criteria present in the literature. Wada et al. (2020) made an important point, commenting that a detailed description of the anatomy remains one of the best ways to better understand the pathophysiology and clinical applicability of myofascial trigger points. Nevertheless, the lack of detailed anatomical information still constitutes a major setback for a complete understanding of the physiopathology and the larger clinical applicability of MTrPs.

Once a trigger point is located, apply firm pressure with the thumbs (Figure 5.29a, Figure 5.29b) or the tip of the elbow (Figure 5.29c). Constant feedback should be sought from the athlete (using a 1–10 pain scale). The level of discomfort should gradually reduce over time (10–30 seconds).

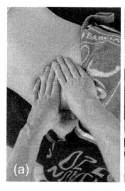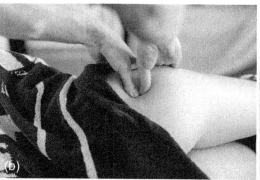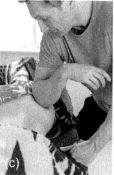

Figure 5.29 (a) Gluteus medius (prone) – thumbs. (b) Gluteals in side-lying – thumbs. (c) Using the elbow.

References

Ajimsha, M.S., Al-Mudahka, N.R. and Al-Madzhar, J.A., 2015. Effectiveness of myofascial release: Systematic review of randomized controlled trials. *Journal of Bodywork and Movement Therapies, 19*(1), pp. 102–112.

Alghadir, A.H., Iqbal, A., Anwer, S., Iqbal, Z.A. and Ahmed, H., 2020. Efficacy of combination therapies on neck pain and muscle tenderness in male patients with upper trapezius active myofascial trigger points. *BioMed Research International, 2020*, p. 9361405. https://doi.org/10.1155/2020/9361405

Amini, A., Goljaryan, S., Shakouri, S.K. and Mohammadimajd, E., 2017. The effects of manual passive muscle shortening and positional release therapy on latent myofascial trigger points of the upper trapezius: A double-blind randomized clinical trial. *Iranian Red Crescent Medical Journal, 19*(9). doi: 10.5812/ircmj.55579

Anderson, A., McConville, A., Fanthorpe, L. and Davis, J., 2017. Salicylate poisoning potential of topical pain relief agents: From age old remedies to engineered smart patches. *Medicines, 4*(3), p. 48.

Arguisuelas, M.D., Lisón, J.F., Sánchez-Zuriaga, D., Martínez-Hurtado, I. and Doménech-Fernández, J., 2017. Effects of myofascial release in nonspecific chronic low back pain: A randomized clinical trial. *Spine, 42*(9), pp. 627–634.

Behm, D.G. and Wilke, J., 2019. Do self-myofascial release devices release myofascia? Rolling mechanisms: A narrative review. *Sports Medicine, 49*(8), pp. 1173–1181.

Benito-de-Pedro, M., Becerro-de-Bengoa-Vallejo, R., Elena Losa-Iglesias, M., Rodríguez-Sanz, D., López-López, D., Palomo-López, P., Mazoteras-Pardo, V. and Calvo-Lobo, A.C., 2020. Effectiveness of deep dry needling vs ischemic compression in the latent myofascial trigger points of the shortened triceps surae from triathletes on ankle dorsiflexion, dynamic, and static plantar pressure distribution: A clinical trial. *Pain Medicine, 21*(2), pp. e172–e181.

Blessing, E.M., Steenkamp, M.M., Manzanares, J. and Marmar, C.R., 2015. Cannabidiol as a potential treatment for anxiety disorders. *Neurotherapeutics, 12*(4), pp. 825–836.

Bookwala, T., Dabholkar, T.Y., Pandit, U., Thakur, A., Karajgi, A. and Yardi, S., 2015. Comparison of efficacy of active release technique with ultrasound and strain-counterstrain technique with ultrasound on upper trapezius trigger points. *Indian Journal of Public Health Research & Development, 6*(3), pp. 264–270.

Cagnie, B., Castelein, B., Pollie, F., Steelant, L., Verhoeyen, H. and Cools, A., 2015. Evidence for the use of ischemic compression and dry needling in the management of trigger points of the upper trapezius in patients with neck pain: A systematic review. *American Journal of Physical Medicine & Rehabilitation, 94*(7), pp. 573–583.

Chaudhry, H., Schleip, R., Ji, Z., Bukiet, B., Maney, M. and Findley, T., 2008. Three-dimensional mathematical model for deformation of human fasciae in manual therapy. *The Journal of the American Osteopathic Association*, *108*(8), pp. 379–390.

Chaudhry, H., Bukiet, B., Ji, Z., Stecco, A. and Findley, T.W., 2014. Deformations experienced in the human skin, adipose tissue, and fascia in osteopathic manipulative medicine. *The Journal of the American Osteopathic Association*, *114*(10), pp. 780–787.

Chen, Q., Bensamoun, S., Basford, J.R., Thompson, J.M. and An, K.N., 2007. Identification and quantification of myofascial taut bands with magnetic resonance elastography. *Archives of Physical Medicine and Rehabilitation*, *88*(12), pp. 1658–1661.

Cyriax, J., 1984. *Textbook of orthopaedic medicine treatment by manipulation, massage and injection.* Vol. *2*. London: Bailliere Tindall.

Davis, J.E., 2007. Are one or two dangerous? Methyl salicylate exposure in toddlers. *The Journal of Emergency Medicine*, *32*(1), pp. 63–69.

Fakhro, M.A., Chahine, H., Srour, H. and Hijazi, K., 2020. Effect of deep transverse friction massage vs stretching on football players' performance. *World Journal of Orthopedics*, *11*(1), p. 47.

Fernández-de-las-Peñas, C. and Dommerholt, J., 2018. International consensus on diagnostic criteria and clinical considerations of myofascial trigger points: A Delphi study. *Pain Medicine*, *19*(1), pp. 142–150.

Field, T., Hernandez-Reif, M., Diego, M., Schanberg, S. and Kuhn, C., 2005. Cortisol decreases and serotonin and dopamine increase following massage therapy. *International Journal of Neuroscience*, *115*(10), pp. 1397–1413.

Gamelin, F.X., Cuvelier, G., Mendes, A., Aucouturier, J., Berthoin, S., Di Marzo, V. and Heyman, E., 2020. Cannabidiol in sport: Ergogenic or else? *Pharmacological Research*, *156*, p. 104764.

Gerez, J.J.G., Figallo, M.Á.S., Martínez, P.V.M., Rabadán, M.F., Ortega, M.Á.L., Vidal, J.A.G. and Hernández, M.S., 2019. Short term application of the muscular inhibition method of strain/counter-strain in the treatment of latent myofascial trigger points of the masticatory musculature: A randomized controlled trial. *Clinical Advances in Health Research*, *1*(1), pp. 2–10.

Hongratanaworakit, T., 2010. Stimulating effect of aromatherapy massage with jasmine oil. *Natural product communications*, *5*(1), p. 1934578X1000500136.

Kage, V. and Ratnam, R., 2014. Immediate effect of active release technique versus mulligan bent leg raise in subjects with hamstring tightness: A randomized clinical trial. *International Journal of Physiotherapy and Research*, *2*(1), pp. 301–304.

Kameda, M. and Tanimae, H., 2019. Effectiveness of active soft tissue release and trigger point block for the diagnosis and treatment of low back and leg pain of predominantly gluteus medius origin: A report of 115 cases. *Journal of Physical Therapy Science*, *31*(2), pp. 141–148.

Kamkaen, N., Ruangrungsi, N., Patalung, N.N. and Watthanachaiyingcharoen, R., 2015. Physiological and psychological effects of lemongrass and sweet almond massage oil. *Journal of Health Research*, *29*(2), pp. 85–91.

Kannabiran, B., 2015. A comparative study of the effectiveness of two manual therapy techniques on pain and lumbar range of motion in individuals with mechanical low back ache. *EC Orthopaedics*, *2*, pp. 36–42.

Kasper, A.M., Sparks, S.A., Hooks, M., Skeer, M., Webb, B., Nia, H., Morton, J.P. and Close, G.L., 2020. High prevalence of cannabidiol use within male professional Rugby Union and League players: A quest for pain relief and enhanced recovery. *International Journal of Sport Nutrition and Exercise Metabolism*, *30*(5), pp. 315–322.

Khan, A., Khan, A.R. and Zafar, M., 2020. Efficacy of Ischemic compression techniques and home exercise programme in combination with US among computer users with upper trapezius myofascial pain. *International Journal of Health Sciences and Research*, *10*(6), pp. 62–67.

Khoshno, H., Mohammadi, F., Dalvandi, A. and Azad, M., 2016. The effect of effleurage massage duration on sleep quality improvement. *Iranian Journal of Rehabilitation Research*, *2*(4), pp. 10–18.

Kidd, R.F., 2009. Why myofascial release will never be evidence-based. *International Musculoskeletal Medicine*, *31*(2), pp. 55–56.

Kim, J.H., Lee, H.S. and Park, S.W., 2015. Effects of the active release technique on pain and range of motion of patients with chronic neck pain. *Journal of Physical Therapy Science*, *27*(8), pp. 2461–2464.

Kligler, B. and Chaudary, S., 2007. Peppermint oil. *American Family Physician*, *75*(7), pp. 1027–1030.

Kraft, K., Kanter, S. and Janik, H., 2013. Safety and effectiveness of vibration massage by deep oscillations: A prospective observational study. *Evidence-Based Complementary and Alternative Medicine*, *2013*, p. 679248. https://doi.org/10.1155/2013/679248

Kumar, G.Y., Sneha, P. and Sivajyothi, N., 2015. Effectiveness of muscle energy technique, Ischaemic compression and strain counter-strain on upper trapezius trigger points: A comparative study. *International Journal of Physical Education, Sports and Health*, *1*(3), pp. 22–26.

Laimi, K., Mäkilä, A., Bärlund, E., Katajapuu, N., Oksanen, A., Seikkula, V., Karppinen, J. and Saltychev, M., 2018. Effectiveness of myofascial release in treatment of chronic musculoskeletal pain: A systematic review. *Clinical Rehabilitation*, *32*(4), pp. 440–450.

Li, L., Stoop, R., Clijsen, R., Hohenauer, E., Fernández-de-Las-Peñas, C., Huang, Q. and Barbero, M., 2020. Criteria used for the diagnosis of myofascial trigger points in clinical trials on physical therapy: Updated systematic review. *The Clinical Journal of Pain*, *36*(12), pp. 955–967.

Mishra, D., Prakash, R.H., Mehta, J. and Dhaduk, A., 2018. Comparative study of active release technique and myofascial release technique in treatment of patients with upper trapezius spasm. *Journal of Clinical & Diagnostic Research*, *12*(11), pp. YC01–4.

Mohamadi, M., Piroozi, S., Rashidi, I. and Hosseinifard, S., 2017. Friction massage versus kinesiotaping for short-term management of latent trigger points in the upper trapezius: A randomized controlled trial. *Chiropractic & Manual Therapies*, *25*(1), pp. 1–6.

Mohamadyari, S., Shojaedin, S.S. and Barati, A.H., 2018. Comparison of two methods of sports massage and cold stretch on the threshold of pain in passive trigger points in shoulder girdle muscles of the female volleyball players. *Journal of Gorgan University of Medical Sciences*, *20*(1), pp. 1–4.

Montañez Aguilera, F.J., Pecos Martín, D., Barrios Pitarque, C., Bosch Morell, F., Valtueña Gimeno, N. and Arnau Masanet, R., 2010. Changes in a patient with neck pain after application of ischemic compression as a trigger point therapy. *Journal of Back and Musculoskeletal Rehabilitation*, *23*(2), pp. 101–104.

Monteiro Rodrigues, L., Rocha, C., Ferreira, H.T. and Silva, H.N., 2020. Lower limb massage in humans increases local perfusion and impacts systemic hemodynamics. *Journal of Applied Physiology*, *128*(5), pp. 1217–1226.

Moraska, A.F., Schmiege, S.J., Mann, J.D., Burtyn, N. and Krutsch, J.P., 2017. Responsiveness of myofascial trigger points to single and multiple trigger point release massages–a randomized, placebo-controlled trial. *American Journal of Physical Medicine & Rehabilitation*, *96*(9), p. 639.

Morihisa, R., Eskew, J., McNamara, A. and Young, J., 2016. Dry needling in subjects with muscular trigger points in the lower quarter: A systematic review. *International Journal of Sports Physical Therapy*, *11*(1), p. 1.

Ogai, R., Yamane, M., Matsumoto, T. and Kosaka, M., 2008. Effects of petrissage massage on fatigue and exercise performance following intensive cycle pedalling. *British Journal of Sports Medicine*, *42*(10), pp. 834–838.

Onik, G., Kasprzyk, T., Knapik, K., Wieczorek, K., Sieroń, D., Sieroń, A., Cholewka, A. and Sieroń, K., 2020. Myofascial trigger points therapy modifies thermal map of Gluteal region. *BioMed Research International*, *2020*, article 4328253. https://doi.org/10.1155/2020/4328253

Paine T., 2000. *The complete guide to sports massage* (Vol. 9, pp. 79–114). London: A & C Black Publishing Ltd.

Palmieri, B., Laurino, C. and Vadalà, M., 2019. A therapeutic effect of cbd-enriched ointment in inflammatory skin diseases and cutaneous scars. *Clinical Therapeutics*, *170*(2), pp. e93–e99.

Paoli, A., Bianco, A., Battaglia, G., Bellafiore, M., Grainer, A., Marcolin, G., Cardoso, C.C., Dall'Aglio, R. and Palma, A., 2013. Sports massage with ozonised oil or non-ozonised oil: Comparative effects on recovery parameters after maximal effort in cyclists. *Physical Therapy in Sport*, *14*(4), pp. 240–245.

Peta, T. and Cardoso, R., 2020. Ischemic compression effects on upper trapezius myofascial trigger points: A systematic review. *International Journal of Public Health Research*, *7*(4), p. 41.

Pitsillides, A. and Stasinopoulos, D., 2019. Cyriax friction massage – Suggestions for improvements. *Medicina*, *55*(5), p. 185.

Reillo, M.R. and Levin, I., 2019. Cannabidiol CBD in the management of sports related traumatic brain injury research and efficacy. *Sports Injuries & Medicine*, *3*, p. 158. doi: 10.29011/2576-9596.100058

Sadria, G., Hosseini, M., Rezasoltani, A., Bagheban, A.A., Davari, A. and Seifolahi, A., 2017. A comparison of the effect of the active release and muscle energy techniques on the latent trigger points of the upper trapezius. *Journal of Bodywork and Movement Therapies*, *21*(4), pp. 920–925.

Schleip, R., 2003a. Fascial plasticity–a new neurobiological explanation: Part 1. *Journal of Bodywork and Movement Therapies*, *7*(1), pp. 11–19.

Schleip, R., 2003b. Fascial plasticity–a new neurobiological explanation Part 2. *Journal of Bodywork and Movement Therapies*, *7*(2), pp. 104–116.

Segura-Ortí, E., Prades-Vergara, S., Manzaneda-Piña, L., Valero-Martínez, R. and Polo-Traverso, J.A., 2016. Trigger point dry needling versus strain-counterstrain technique for upper trapezius myofascial trigger points: A randomised controlled trial. *Acupuncture in Medicine*, *34*(3), pp. 171–177.

Shah, S. and Bhalara, A., 2012. Myofascial release. *International Journal of Health Sciences and Research*, *2*(2), pp. 69–77.

Shokri, E., Mohamadi, M. and Heidari, S., 2015. Treatment of myofascial trigger points of pelvic floor with physiotherapeutic package: A case report. *Journal of Rehabilitation Sciences & Research*, *2*(1), pp. 20–22.

Silva, J., Abebe, W., Sousa, S.M., Duarte, V.G., Machado, M.I.L. and Matos, F.J.A., 2003. Analgesic and anti-inflammatory effects of essential oils of Eucalyptus. *Journal of Ethnopharmacology*, *89*(2–3), pp. 277–283.

Sullivan, K.M., Silvey, D.B., Button, D.C. and Behm, D.G., 2013. Roller-massager application to the hamstrings increases sit-and-reach range of motion within five to ten seconds without performance impairments. *International Journal of Sports Physical Therapy*, *8*(3), p. 228.

Takamoto, K., Bito, I., Urakawa, S., Sakai, S., Kigawa, M., Ono, T. and Nishijo, H., 2015. Effects of compression at myofascial trigger points in patients with acute low back pain: A randomized controlled trial. *European Journal of Pain*, *19*(8), pp. 1186–1196.

Threlkeld, A.J., 1992. The effects of manual therapy on connective tissue. *Physical Therapy*, *72*(12), pp. 893–902.

Trivedi, P., Sathiyavani, D., Nambi, G., Khuman, R., Shah, K. and Bhatt, P., 2014. Comparison of active release technique and myofascial release technique on pain, grip strength & functional performance in patients with chronic lateral epicondylitis. *International Journal of Physiotherapy and Research*, *2*(3), pp. 488–494.

Trivedi, P., Bhatt, P., Dhanakotti, S. and Nambi, G., 2016. Comparison of muscle energy technique and myofascial release technique on pain and range of motion in patients with temporomandibular joint dysfunction: A randomized controlled study. *International Journal of Physiotherapy and Research*, *4*(6), pp. 1788–1792.

Vijayakumar, M., Jaideep, A. and Khankal, R., 2019. Effectiveness of compressive myofascial release vs instrument assisted soft tissue mobilization in subjects with active trigger points of the calf muscle limiting ankle dorsiflexion. *International Journal of Health Sciences and Research*, *9*(4), pp. 98–106.

Wada, J.T., Akamatsu, F., Hojaij, F., Itezerote, A., Scarpa, J.C., Andrade, M. and Jacomo, A., 2020. An anatomical basis for the myofascial trigger points of the abductor hallucis muscle. *BioMed Research International*, *2020*, p. 9240581. doi:10.1155/2F2020/2F9240581

Wong, C.K., Abraham, T., Karimi, P. and Ow-Wing, C., 2014. Strain counter-strain technique to decrease tender point palpation pain compared to control conditions: A systematic review with meta-analysis. *Journal of Bodywork and Movement Therapies, 18*(2), pp. 165–173.

Wong, R.W.K. and Rabie, A.B.M., 2008. Local massage with topical analgesic, a novel treatment modality for temporomandibular muscular pain, a case study report of 5 consecutive cases. *The Open Orthopaedics Journal, 2*, p. 97.

World Anti-Doping Agency, 2013. *New threshold level for Cannabis.* Montreal, QC, Canada: WADA.

Xu, D.H., Cullen, B.D., Tang, M. and Fang, Y., 2020. The Effectiveness of topical cannabidiol oil in symptomatic relief of peripheral neuropathy of the lower extremities. *Current Pharmaceutical Biotechnology, 21*(5), pp. 390–402.

Zein-Hammoud, M. and Standley, P.R., 2015. Modeled osteopathic manipulative treatments: a review of their in vitro effects on fibroblast tissue preparations. *The Journal of the American Osteopathic Association, 115*(8), pp. 490–502.

Zhong, H., Wang, C., Wan, Z. and Lei, J., 2019. The techniques of manual massage and its application on exercise-induced fatigue: A literature review. *Frontiers in Sport Research, 1*(1), pp. 43–50.

6 The Effects of Massage on Sports Performance

Massage Prior to Athletic Performance

A number of studies have examined the effects of pre-performance massage on sprint performance in college-based athletes (Goodwin et al., 2007; Arabaci, 2008; Fletcher, 2010; Arazi et al., 2012; Moran et al., 2018). For example, Fletcher (2010) investigated the kinematic parameters of sprint performance following nine minutes of lower-limb massage, a traditional warm up and a pre-competition massage and a traditional warm up (4 × 20-metre strides were also added to the massage intervention group prior to the sprint performance). The active warm up condition resulted in a 2.74% significant reduction in sprint time when compared to the massage only condition. The author concluded that the decrease in step rate and knee velocity observed after massage could be the result of a reduction in discharge from the muscle spindles due to increased muscle compliance. However, it should be noted when massage was combined with an active warm up, no significant differences were found. Goodwin and colleagues (2007) included 37 university students, all completing three 30-metre sprints with five-minute rest intervals between the sprints. Their results indicated that 15 minutes of massage had no significant effect on sprint performance; however, this is unsurprising, as following the massage the participants completed a 10-minute active warm up, had 5 minutes of recovery and had 5-minute breaks between the sprints. It is also worth noting that three different massage therapists were used in this study, which also may have confounded their results. These two investigations concluded that pre-performance massage is likely to have a neutral (Goodwin et al., 2007) or detrimental effect on sprint performance unless combined with an active warm up, could potentially be a waste of time and money and therefore should not be seen as an important part of a warm up (Fletcher, 2010). In addition, 17 collegiate sprinters received 10–15 minutes of stimulatory massage by a licenced athletic trainer prior to completing 20-, 30- and 60-metre sprints (Moran et al., 2018). In this study the authors compared four treatment conditions including pre-competition stimulatory massage, dynamic warm up, a combination of massage and warm up, and placebo ultrasound. The research did not state the stroke rate used in the massage protocol, so the definition of a 'stimulatory' massage should be interpreted cautiously. The results indicated no significant differences in acceleration and sprint performance between the four interventions. This led the authors to conclude that the use of a pre-competition massage as a warm-up modality, whether alone or combined with a dynamic warm-up, has no benefit to enhancing acceleration and sprint performance.

Investigating the difference between warm-up massage, an active warm up, and no warm up on an agility test (T-test), rates of perceived exertion (RPE) and a sit and reach test in high-level amateur tennis players, Bedford and colleagues (2018) indicated 5 minutes of stimulatory massage (120 strokes/circles per minute) had no statistically significant physiological

DOI: 10.4324/9781003104803-6

performance effects, but there was a small reduction in the rate of perceived exertion (RPE) in the massage group compared to the no warm up group ($p < 0.001$), demonstrating passive warming up (massage) could have a small psychological benefit. Both warm-up interventions also demonstrated improvements in hip flexion range of motion (sit and reach), possibly as a result of increased tissue temperature or altered neural mechanisms.

In similar studies by Arabaci (2008) and Arazi et al. (2012) using male college students, vertical jump height (VJ) and sprint performances were analysed following 15 minutes of lower-limb massage. The results from Arazi et al.'s study showed a significant worsening in VJ, 10-, 20- and 30-metre sprint and T-test times following massage. There were no significant changes in the rest (control) group. These results concur with those reported by Arabaci (2008) who also found massage following an active warm up significantly degraded performance in VJ, 10-metre acceleration, a flying start 20-metre sprint and a 30-metre sprint from a standing position, possibly due to a reduction in muscle stiffness and associated neural mechanisms. Two massage therapists were used to deliver the intervention, leading to the possibility the massage techniques may have been applied differently. Another study, conducted by Arroyo-Morrales and colleagues (2011) and using a randomised single-blind placebo-controlled crossover design, compared the effects of 20 minutes of leg massage and sham ultrasound as a control condition on isokinetic peak torque. The authors suggested that massage has a detrimental effect on peak torque as a result of decreased motor unit activation, but this applied solely to the quadriceps at speed of $240°/s$ and $180°/s$. There were no significant interactions at speeds of $120°/s$ and $60°/s$, or for any mean peak torque values in the knee flexors (hamstrings). Vertical jump height and a 4×9-metre running test carrying a wooden block (performed twice) were analysed in a poorly designed study by Mustafaloo (2012). The participants received a 15-minute lower body massage prior to the performance task, in one of the few studies to use high-level football players. In their running and vertical jump height tests, no significant performance differences were found following massage.

The only study (McKetchnie et al., 2007) to compare two different types of massage, vigorous petrissage and tapotement, prior to participants performing a drop jump and concentric calf raise, was conducted in a well-designed study using male and female participants who each received three minutes of massage to the plantar flexors prior to two tests of muscle power. The authors' statistical analysis revealed that there were no significant differences between the conditions in any of the variables related to power or the concentric calf raise. The researchers noted the possibility of any positive effect of massage on the neural system counterbalancing or eliminating the negative effects of increased muscle compliance. Moreover, other equivocal findings within the literature have been found; for example, Hunter et al. (2006) noted a decrement in force production at $60°/s$ after a 20-minute massage intervention, and a near significant decrement at $120°/s$. However, no decrements were found at speeds of 180 and $240°/s$, or in vertical jump height.

The majority of studies on massage prior to performance have concentrated on the lower body, but equivocal findings have also been found in studies on massage prior to tests of grip strength. Short duration massage of 3 minutes (Bedford & Robbins, 2016), and longer durations of 15 minutes (Khamwong et al., 2010) have demonstrated no beneficial performance outcomes in grip strength. In contrast, Brooks et al. (2005) found 5 minutes of massage to the forearm musculature improved post-exercise grip performance, which they concluded could be as a result of increased temperature and blood flow. These findings were in agreement with those of Molouki et al. (2016) who noted improvements to grip strength (although not significantly) and grip endurance in a group of 44 healthy young men immediately after one session of massage to the forearm and hand.

In summary, results indicate that massage prior to athletic performance or in conjunction with an active warm-up routine is likely to have detrimental (Arabaci, 2008; Arazi et al., 2012), mixed (Fletcher, 2010; Arroyo-Morrales et al., 2011), neutral (Goodwin et al., 2007; McKetchnie et al., 2007; Bedford & Robbins, 2016; Bedford et al., 2018) or positive results on athletic performance (Brooks et al., 2005; Molouki et al., 2016). As massage stimulates sensory afferent fibres in the skin (Sarli & Agus, 2014), pre-competition massage may provide some short-term pain relief when required and may offer other psychological benefits. However, physiologically, no increased performance enhancement is likely, according to the majority of the current evidence on lower body explosive type movement. It should be noted that the wide range in research methodology and poorly controlled studies, including different stroke rates, length of massage, pressure administered and techniques used (Paine, 2000; Caldwell, 2001; McKetchnie et al., 2007; Arazi et al., 2012) does make results difficult to interpret. Given the huge number of potential massage regimens and timings, it is impossible to conclude that massage cannot improve performance if the correct timing and indication could be defined (Davis et al., 2020).

When warming up the calf area, the foot should be stabilised (see Figure 6.1). Both hands work alternately at a fast rate (120 strokes per minute) in an upward direction, to generate as

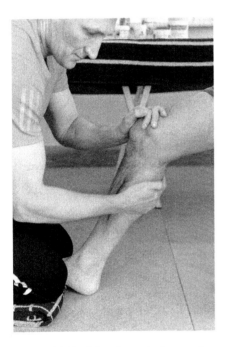

Figure 6.1 Both hands work alternately at a fast rate in an upward direction.

much heat as possible in the muscle. If the athlete's knee moves too much laterally when massaging the calf or hamstring, stabilise the foot or knee with one hand to avoid excessive movement, and swap hands as necessary (Figure 6.2).

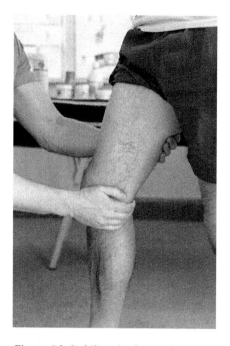

Figure 6.2 Stabilise the foot or knee to avoid excessive movement with one hand, and swap hands as necessary.

When warming up the lower back (Figure 6.3) always protect the athlete's clothing (especially if topical heat lotions are being used). Work in large circular motions covering all the musculature until all the cream/lotion has absorbed into the skin.

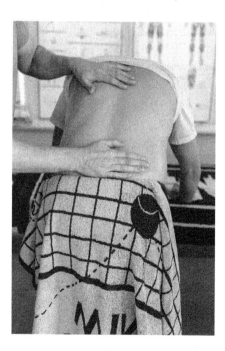

Figure 6.3 Protect the athletes clothing (especially if topical heat lotions are being used).

The left hand works on the upper trapezius and posterior aspect of the shoulder whilst the right hand works on the pectoral, anterior deltoid and upper bicep, with the thumbs covering the medial deltoid (Figure 6.4). All of the palmar aspect of the hand is used on the athlete's shoulder. To minimise therapist fatigue, where possible have the athlete in a seated position.

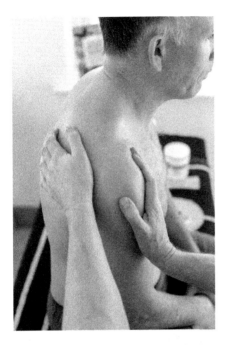

Figure 6.4 The left hand covers the upper trapezius and posterior aspect of the shoulder. The right hand covers on the pectoral, anterior deltoid, and upper bicep. Use the thumbs over the medial deltoid.

The Effect of Massage on Female Athletes

Dariusz and colleagues (2014) compared the effects of eight minutes of massage (four on each leg) on 59 women prior to a long jump test from standing, a 10-second run on the spot with hand claps, and 30 squats in 30 seconds (Ruffier test). This study had a number of methodological flaws, but refreshingly it did compare different ages and exercise experiences in the females attending aerobic classes. Standard warm up without massage proved to be the least effective across the performance measures in all tests. Interestingly, massage had a greater impact on women under the age of 30 with little exercise experience. In those with greater experience, massage appeared to have a reduced benefit, particularly in the power and speed tests. In another study of 29 women aged 24–26 (Boguszewski et al., 2014), the participants performed five sets of deep squats to induce muscle soreness. Exercise intensity was measured using Borg's ratings of perceived exertion scale (RPE), and a visual analogue scale (VAS) was used to assess muscle soreness levels at 24, 48, 72 and 96 hours after exercise. The results indicated that the largest decrease in lower limb power (vertical jump test) was between the first measurement after the exercise session and 24 hours later ($p < 0.01$). The smallest decrease in power, tested via the vertical jump test, was in the massage group ($n=15$) with the highest levels of muscle soreness noted 24 hours post-exercise in the massage group and 48 hours post-exercise in the control group, who received no treatment (*n*=14). And finally, Mancinelli et al., (2006) found a thigh massage decreased perceived soreness (using pressure pain algometry) and increased vertical jump displacement in a sample of 22 female collegiate basketball and volleyball players, leading the authors to support the use of massage in female collegiate athletes.

It would be interesting if future research compared the same massage protocols (including depth, duration and stroke rate) on a large sample of both male and female athletes, to ascertain if pre- or post-training performance and/or recovery massage had any greater effects on one particular gender.

The Effects of Massage on Delayed Onset Muscle Soreness

Exercise-induced muscle damage (EIMD) is characterised by the delayed onset of muscle soreness (DOMS), often experienced after unfamiliar exercise that produces an increased load or demand, particularly with eccentric contractions (Kalman et al., 2018). Symptoms peak within 24–48 hours (Macintyre et al., 2001; Connolly et al., 2003; Howartson & van Someren, 2008) and subside 5–7 days post-exercise (Khamwong et al., 2010; Lewis et al., 2012). As DOMS is likely to affect physical performance, it is of utmost importance, especially in the field of professional sports, that athletes can be immediately relieved of pain so that they can be trained or compete with the absence of such conditions (Visconti et al., 2020).

It has been suggested that pain experienced during DOMS is a result of lactic acid, muscle spasm, connective tissue damage, muscle damage, inflammation and the enzyme efflux theory (Cheung et al., 2003) with the addition of the mechanical disruption of sarcomeres leading to the inflammatory response, swelling of damaged muscle fibres and the subsequent release of biomarkers such as lactate, ammonia and oxypurines (Shin & Sung, 2015). The associated muscle spasm has also been found to stimulate pain receptors, causing an ischaemic response (Hall, 2010). However, the exact mechanisms behind the development of pain and explanations for its delayed response are still not fully understood, thus no theory has been fully accepted. As swelling is seen to contribute to pain receptor activation (Weerapong et al., 2005), modalities which promote fluid flow would be expected to reduce soreness levels. Visconti et al. (2015) found DOMS responds to massage but does not appear to respond to other modalities such as rest, suggesting an intervention that results in repeated stimulation of afferent nerve endings and nociceptors creates an analgesic response. It is hypothesised that massage involves mechanical pressures leading to an increase in blood and lymph flow, reducing ischemia and fluid accumulation (Black et al., 2003; Veqar & Kalra, 2013), which may help to reduce DOMS-related pain.

Numerous research articles have found massage has a positive effect on reducing DOMS (Farr et al., 2002; Zainuddin et al., 2005; Mancinelli et al., 2006; Law et al., 2008; Boguszewski et al., 2014; Shin & Sung, 2015; Guo et al., 2017; Holub & Smith, 2017; Dupuy et al., 2018). However, others disagree, including Hart and colleagues (2005), who discovered a 5-minute massage to the lower leg after eccentric exercise was not effective in reducing pain levels within 72 hours. They also stated that five minutes of massage did not alter the time course effects of DOMS. In agreement, Dawson et al. (2004) found 30 minutes massage did not affect the recovery measures of strength, swelling or soreness in 12 recreational runners following a half marathon, although the runners did perceive there had been some benefit. Khamwong and colleagues' later study (2010) found a 15-minute massage, pre-exercise, had no significant effect on muscle soreness. Although the authors did find a significant difference in passive ROM, as pain reduced during passive flexion. In addition, Visconti et al. (2020) indicated that neither a 10-minute pain-free effleurage massage, long wave-diathermy nor sham long-wave diathermy (placebo) had any significant effect in relieving DOMS (according to a numerical pain rating scale). However, in the massage group the participants generally reported feeling 'better' or 'moderately better' after receiving the treatment, highlighting that massage may have a positive psychological influence on perceived pain from DOMS rather than a physiological one.

A number of variables need to be considered when comparing studies. For example, results may be limited by the target muscles used, the application time, techniques used, stroke rates administered, and potentially the most important aspect, duration of treatment (Khamwong et al., 2010). Kargarfard et al. (2016) used 30 male bodybuilders, each receiving 30 minutes of sports massage following strenuous exercise. Plasma creatine kinase (CK) level, an agility test, vertical jump test, isometric torque test and perception of soreness were all analysed immediately following massage and at 24, 48 and 72 hours after massage. Both groups showed significant ($p < 0.001$) decreases in jumping, agility performance and isometric torque, but significant ($p < 0.001$) increases in CK and muscle soreness levels. However, the authors noted that the massage group generally demonstrated a better recovery rate.

Massage of the gastrocnemius muscle after exercise-induced muscle damage (EIMD) improved muscle strength and proprioception by influencing the superficial (but not in the deep) muscle layers in a study by Shin and Sung (2015). The timing and method of massage used in this experiment may have affected muscle fibre regeneration, with the authors speculating that this change may be a result of the mechanical action of massage promoting a return to normal muscle fibre alignment. Therefore, these findings demonstrate that massage for EIMD can improve proprioceptive accuracy and muscle strength. A systematic review (28 trials) on the efficacy of manual massage versus local vibratory massage, promoting recovery from exercise-induced muscle damage, was conducted by Ntshangase and Peters-Futre (2017). The authors concluded that most studies had methodological flaws, but manual massage was no more effective than local vibratory massage in controlling functional decline from exercise-induced muscle damage. In another systematic review by Guo et al. (2017) the authors summarised that massage as an intervention could be effective for alleviating DOMS as well as increasing muscle performance after strenuous exercise. The highest efficacy was achieved at 48 hours post-exercise. However, the authors went on to highlight that caution should be taken when interpreting results due to sample sizes and limitations within their reviewed studies. Finally, the results from a study by Imtiyaz et al. (2014) indicated that vibration therapy (50Hz for 5 minutes) and massage therapy (15 minutes) are both equally effective in the prevention of DOMS. Massage is more effective in restoration of concentric strength (1 RM), yet vibration therapy shows clinically an early reduction in pain and is effective in decreasing the level of lactate dehydrogenase 48 hours post-exercise periods.

Does Massage Increase Blood Flow and Temperature?

It is reasonable to suggest that the rubbing action of massage across the surface of the skin could have a superficial effect on blood flow and create an increase in local tissue temperature. This point was demonstrated by Sefton and his associates (2010) who suggested their 20-minute massage protocol could increase skin and peripheral blood perfusion to the area receiving massage, as well as to adjacent areas. They also speculated that a prolonged increase in temperature may influence the oxygen/haemoglobin dissociation curve, resulting in the delivery of oxygen to the tissues. In another study (Mori et al., 2004), muscle blood volume and skin temperature were both shown to increase (0.45°C) in the lumbar muscle region in 29 volunteers following 5 minutes of massage. However, the authors concluded this could have been from the massage or heat conduction from the therapist's hands. In an investigation in 2003,

Drust and colleagues evaluated the effects of different durations of deep effleurage massage of the vastus lateralis, measuring intra-muscular temperature at depths of 1.5, 2.5 and 3.5 cms. The authors found significantly greater changes in muscle temperature at 1.5 and 2.5 cms following massage (2–3°C).

Hinds and co-authors highlighted an important point in 2004, indicating that without an increase in arterial blood flow, any increase in skin blood flow potentially diverts blood flow away from the recovering muscle, and therefore could potentially have the opposite desired effect.

Furthermore, in a study by Wiltshire and colleagues (2010), blood flow to the forearm muscle was impaired by massage during the first 4.5 minutes of recovery following intense forearm exercise. Interestingly, lactic acid efflux was also reduced by massage as a direct impairment of forearm blood flow (25% over 10.5 minutes of recovery) leading the authors to recommend that sports massage should not be indicated for removal of lactic acid from exercised muscle. Shah et al.'s (2017) study demonstrated that integrated myofascial techniques increased peripheral blood flow in the paraspinal muscles in 44 healthy participants when compared to Kinesio tape and sham TENS (placebo). However, this had no beneficial effect in pain responses, highlighting increasing peripheral blood flow has no impact on pain outcomes.

The Psychological Effects of Massage

Laux et al.'s 2015 study made an interesting association between the feeling of muscles being stiff and the feeling of being prone to injury. These factors also fit the assumption of the stress and injury model which proposes generalised muscle tension and fear of injury to be important mediating factors between stress and injury. Therefore, the physiological and psychological benefit of including massage as part of specific muscle injury treatment to help relieve tightness, reduce fatigue, or reduce perceptions of tightness and fatigue should not be overlooked. The injury cycle is shown in Figure 6.5.

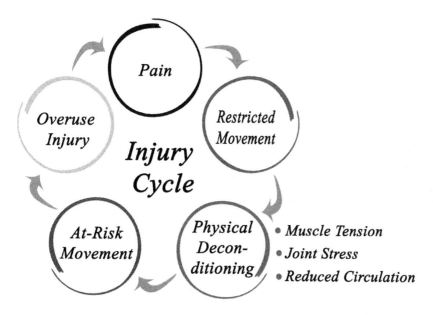

Figure 6.5 Pain cycle: physiology and psychology.

Pain reduction may well be a psychological concept, and any analgesic effects of massage may therefore be due to the athlete's individual expectations of treatment and their own individual modulation in regard to pain. Zusman (2013) found positive communication such as 'because you are unable to move about normally, to get you started I am going to use my hands to help your back to move properly. We are greatly assisted in this regard by the fact that when skillfully applied the treatment I use directly inhibits pain'.

Therefore, it is unclear whether the effects of manual therapy are solely physiological or are in fact more psychological when effectively measuring perceived amounts of pain or discomfort, particularly if massage is accompanied by positive reinforcement.

Furthermore, a number of studies have reported that massage has beneficial outcomes on pain and perceived fatigue. For instance, Nunes and colleagues (2016) reported relief of symptoms following 7 minutes of massage to the quadriceps in 74 athletes following a long-distance Ironman triathlon. Hemmings et al. (2000) found evidence of psychological regeneration (using a perceived recovery scale) following massage during the recovery phase of repeated sports performance in amateur boxers. These results also agree with Szabo and colleagues (2008), who discovered 10 minutes of pre-event massage significantly lowered perceived exertion scores in female runners. Delextrat et al. (2013) compared the effects of massage and intermittent cold-water immersion in male and female basketball players following competitive matches. There was lower perception of fatigue overall, and in the legs specifically, immediately after the massage and cold-water immersion condition ($p < 0.001$). Interestingly women had a lower perception of fatigue in cold-water immersion compared to massage at any testing time ($p < 0.001$), with no effect from any of the recovery interventions on repeated-sprint measures (p at best 0.067). Therefore, aside from repeated sprinting, these results suggest both massage and cold-water immersion improve perceptual measures of recovery. In addition, wrestlers receiving 25 minutes of massage over ten sessions (Zadkhosh et al., 2015) demonstrated decreased depression ($p < 0.001$), anxiety ($p < 0.001$) and stress ($p < 0.001$) scores, compared to experimental and control groups.

Other studies have demonstrated lower anxiety, lower cortisol levels and improved profile of mood state questionnaire scores (POMS) in female dancers (Leivadi et al., 1999) and cyclists (Micklewright et al., 2005) following their respective massage interventions. In addition, men who received two massages within 2 weeks prior to an aerobic sports event felt massage was relaxing, and they perceived there to be a reduction in stress, a decrease in nervous tension and anxiety, and improved concentration. Physiologically, they felt massage reduced muscle stiffness, they had less cramping and soreness and had less trouble from previous injuries (Jooste et al., 2013). An investigation using para-athletes, including seven male and two female participants of the Roger C Peace paracycling team ($n = 9$), completed questionnaires over a 6-month period using 10-point scales for pain, sleep, function, spasticity and stress before, during and after a massage intervention. The athletes reported an improvement in muscular tension and sleep after the massage treatment and felt it helped with recovery and training, but it did not significantly improve quality of life as measured by the SF-36 instruments and did not significantly improve pain or stress levels (Kennedy et al., 2018).

Does Massage Increase Range of Motion?

The possibility of massage increasing flexibility has been investigated with mixed results. Research into hip flexion range of motion, using a sit and reach test following massage to the hamstrings, demonstrated that individuals with already tighter hamstrings showed the most improvement, with an increase in hamstring flexibility of 4.7 degrees following dynamic soft tissue techniques (Hopper et al., 2005). By contrast, Barlow and colleagues (2004) found no increase in hamstring flexibility (sit and reach test) following a single 15-minute session of massage. However, Arabaci (2008) and Bedford et al. (2018) noted an improvement in hamstring flexibility, again using the sit and reach test, after 15 minutes (of which 10 minutes was to the posterior limbs) and 5 minutes of massage, respectively. Additionally, positive effects were also found after 30 seconds of massage to the musculotendinous unit, which increased hip flexion by 7.2% in 10 recreationally active women (Huang et al., 2010). In a more recent study by Kaur and Sinha (2020), the authors concluded that Swedish massage acutely increased flexibility of the hamstrings following 7 minutes of massage on each posterior thigh for 5 continuous days, followed by 5 days of no massage. Moreover, the increased flexibility persisted for the 5 days after cessation of massage, making this is one of the few studies to examine the carry-over effects of massage. The majority of studies address lower body flexibility, but a systematic review and meta-analysis (Yeun, 2017) investigating the effectiveness of massage on shoulder range of motion ($n = 237$) suggested that there is evidence of the efficiency of massage therapy for improving shoulder range of motion, particularly flexion and abduction. The increase in range of motion frequently demonstrated in all of the above studies could be as a result of the increase in tissue temperature or altered reflex sensitivity (Bedford et al., 2018).

The Effects of Massage on Recovery

Exercise training at high intensities can induce temporary damage to muscle, with a change in the sarcomeres and components of the excitation-contraction coupling system. Massage reduces mechanical overload on sarcomeres during lengthening actions (eccentric exercise) and prevents sarcoplasmic reticulum ruptures, which decreases intracellular calcium and triggers calcium-sensitive degradative pathways, leading to less ultrastructural damage (Weerapong et al., 2005). Additionally, massage has been hypothesised to moderate inflammation, improve blood flow and reduce tissue stiffness, resulting in a diminished sensation of pain (Crane et al., 2012). It may also be an appropriate counter to fatigue onset due to an ability to influence fluid movement in deep tissue, thereby improving nutrient flow or waste removal, or by facilitating relaxation to promote normal recovery (Morasaka, 2005).

Crane et al.'s 2012 study took biopsies from 11 participants and found that, despite having no effect on muscle metabolites (glycogen, lactate), massage attenuated the production of the inflammatory cytokines tumour necrosis factor-α (TNF-α) and interleukin-6 (IL-6) and reduced heat shock protein 27 (HSP27) phosphorylation, thereby mitigating cellular stress resulting from myofiber injury. These physiological benefits (due to 10 minutes of massage) that modulate protein synthesis, glucose uptake and immune cell recruitment are likely to be initiated through mechanical effects on skeletal muscle, followed by changes to intracellular regulatory cascades. Therefore, from this well-conducted study, it appears that massage is beneficial following muscle damage as a result of strenuous exercise because it reduces inflammation and promotes mitochondrial biogenesis.

During the continual turnover of lactate during active recovery, muscle fibres maintain a concentration gradient that continually draws lactate across the sarcolemma from the extracellular fluid, thus gradually depleting the levels of lactate in the general circulation (Micklewright et al., 2006). Massage involves applying mechanical forces to the active muscles, which potentially increases intracellular hydrostatic pressure. The subsequent effect on the balance between hydrostatic and colloid osmotic pressures enhances the diffusion potential across the sarcolemma, thereby promoting rapid evacuation of lactate from the cell into the extracellular space. Consequently, massage may increase the availability of lactate for gluconeogenesis and oxidative utilisation at other sites of uptake during the early stages of recovery (Micklewright et al., 2006).

Active recovery has been shown to be more effective than massage, and massage more effective than passive recovery, in removing blood lactate in 17 professional male swimmers (Rasooli et al., 2012). In the authors' results, they noted blood lactate decreased after active recovery, massage and passive recovery (blood lactate mean ± SD: 5.72 ± 1.44, 7.10 ± 1.27, 10.94 ± 2.05 mmol/L, respectively). Active and massage recovery ($p = 1.00$) were more effective in improving swimming performance (200 metres separated by 10-minute intervals) than passive recovery. However, Cè et al. (2013) found both deep and superficial massage did not alter La⁻ kinetics compared to passive recovery during maximum voluntary contraction (MVC) of the knee extensor muscles ($n = 9$). These findings indicate that the pressure exerted during massage administration did not play a significant role in post-exercise blood La⁻ levels.

On a negative note, Pinar et al. (2012) used two different therapists to perform their well-described massage protocol (although using two therapists does make standardised massage depth harder to control). Following exhausting exercise (anaerobic Wingate test), no significant differences were found between their interventions (massage, passive rest, electrical muscle stimulation) in heart rate levels, blood lactate concentration ($p = 0.817$, $p = 0.493$, respectively) and rate of perceived exertion levels. By contrast, Dunabeitia et al. (2019) recruited 48 well-trained male runners and compared massage and cold-water immersion (CWI) following an exhaustive interval running session. After repeating the test 48 hours later the massage group had significantly better recovery than the control group at 14 km/h in running economy (RE) ($p < 0.05$; $\eta = 0.176$) and greater stride height and angle changes at 16 km/h ($p < 0.05$; $\eta = 0.166$ and $p < 0.05$; $\eta = 0.208$, respectively). No differences were observed between the CWI and control groups. These results indicate massage to be a superior choice compared to CWI for faster recovery and running biomechanics. Additionally, Romadhona et al. (2019) reported that in recovery using sports massage ($p = 0.001$), and when sports massage is combined with cold water immersion (15°C) ($p = 0.000$), blood lactate levels are reduced following submaximal physical exercise.

Forty-five healthy female non-athletic subjects were recruited and randomly distributed into three groups (15 subjects in each group) in a study by Imtiyaz et al. (2014). In this study, each group received vibration therapy (50 Hz vibration for 5 minutes) or massage therapy (15 minutes), with the control group receiving no treatment, prior to the eccentric exercise protocol (elbow flexors). The authors measured changes in the muscle condition, muscle soreness (pain perception), range of motion (ROM), maximum isometric force (MIF), repetition maximum (RM), lactate dehydrogenase (LDH) and creatine kinase (CK) level. All the parameters except LDH, CK and 1 RM were measured before and immediately post-intervention, immediately post-exercise, and then at 24 hours, 48 hours and 72 hours post-exercise. LDH, CK and 1 RM were measured before and 48 hours post-exercise. This study indicated that vibration therapy and massage therapy are equally effective in prevention of DOMS. Massage proved to be more effective in restoration of concentric strength (1 RM) ($p = 0.000$), yet vibration therapy showed a clinically early reduction of pain and is effective in decreasing the level of LDH 48 hours post-exercise ($p = 0.000$).

A 7-minute massage protocol was performed by Eriksson Crommert et al. (2015) on 18 healthy volunteers to evaluate the effect of massage on stiffness of the medial gastrocnemius (MG) muscle, and to determine whether its effect (if any) persists over a short rest period. The authors measured muscle shear elastic modulus (stiffness) bilaterally (control and massaged leg). Directly following massage, participants rated pain experienced during the massage. MG shear elastic modulus of the massaged leg decreased significantly at follow-up 1 (−5.2 ± 8.8%, $p = 0.019$, $d = −0.66$). There was no difference between follow-up 2 and baseline for the massaged leg ($p = 0.83$), indicating muscle stiffness returned to baseline values immediately after the massage has ceased.

A systematic review by Best et al. (2008) on the efficacy of sports massage for recovery of skeletal muscle from strenuous exercise concluded that the beneficial effects of massage on muscle recovery were best realised when the treatment was administered within two hours of exercise (from six reviewed studies). However, the authors noted in their discussion that when measuring 'recovery', studies varied tremendously in their use of massage type, number of times massage was administered, duration, magnitude, rate and the vast amount of outcome measures. Therefore, it can be concluded that the effects of sports massage on recovery from strenuous exercise still needs further investigation. There are a high number of variables which determine whether massage is likely to be effective, including but not limited to the level of fatigue, amount of muscle trauma induced, timing of massage, depth and duration of treatment, techniques used and athlete perception.

The Effects of Massage on Stress and Anxiety

Noto et al. (2010) reported that salivary cortisol levels did not change after back massage in young healthy females. In addition, Moyer and colleagues' quantitative review (2011) of six reviews found that the effects of massage on cortisol levels proved non-significant or not distinguishable from zero. However, contrary to this, 15-minute doses of massage every day for one week did decrease cortisol levels ($p < 0.05$), state of anxiety ($p < 0.001$) and systolic/diastolic blood pressure ($p < 0.001$/$p < 0.01$ respectively) in a study by Pinar and Afsar (2016). Also, 25 minutes of sports massage reduced stress and anxiety in 15–18-year-old wrestlers (anxiety $p < 0.001$; stress $p < 0.001$), compared to their control group, in a study by Zadkhosh et al. (2015). In addition, the effects of massage therapy on biochemistry (including decreased levels of cortisol and increased levels of serotonin and dopamine) were reviewed by Field et al. (2005). Although this study was not aimed at the athletic community, an average increase of 31% was noted for dopamine, significant decreases were noted in cortisol levels (averaging decreases 31%) and an average increase of 28% was noted for serotonin. From these studies it does appears there is likely to be more of an individual response to markers of stress and anxiety following massage, possibly as a response to other external factors such as trust and rapport built with the therapist. However, during competitive phases where athletes are under high levels of stress, some may find massage a useful tool to reduce pre-competition stress and anxiety.

References

Arabaci, R., 2008. Acute effects of pre-event lower limb massage on explosive and high- speed motor capacities and flexibility. *Journal of Sports Science & Medicine*, 7(4), p. 549.

Arazi, H., Asadi, A. and Hoseini, K., 2012. Comparison of two different warm-ups (static-stretching and massage): Effects on flexibility and explosive power. *Acta Kinesiologica*, 6(1), pp. 55–59.

Arroyo-Morales, M., Fernández-Lao, C., Ariza-García, A., Toro-Velasco, C., Winters, M., Díaz-Rodríguez, L., Cantarero-Villanueva, I., Huijbregts, P. and Fernández-De-las-Peñas, C., 2011. Psychophysiological effects of preperformance massage before isokinetic exercise. *The Journal of Strength & Conditioning Research*, 25(2), pp. 481–488.

Barlow, A., Clarke, R., Johnson, N., Seabourne, B., Thomas, D. and Gal, J., 2004. Effect of massage of the hamstring muscle group on performance of the sit and reach test. *British Journal of Sports Medicine*, 38(3), pp. 349–351.

Bedford, S. and Robbins, D., 2016. The acute effects of massage are not detrimental to grip strength in sub-elite racquet players. *Medicine & Science in Tennis*, 21(1), pp. 24–27.

Bedford, S., Robbins, D. and Fletcher, I., 2018. Effects of an active warm up and warm up massage on agility, perceived exertion, and flexibility in tennis players. *Medicine & Science in Tennis, 3*(2), pp. 16–22.

Best, T.M., Hunter, R., Wilcox, A. and Haq, F., 2008. Effectiveness of sports massage for recovery of skeletal muscle from strenuous exercise. *Clinical Journal of Sport Medicine, 18*(5), pp. 446–460.

Black, C.D., Vickerson, B. and McCully, K.K., 2003. Noninvasive assessment of vascular function in the posterior tibial artery of healthy humans. *Dynamic Medicine, 2*(1), pp. 1–7.

Boguszewski, D., Szkoda, S., Adamczyk, J.G. and Białoszewski, D., 2014. Sports massage therapy on the reduction of delayed onset muscle soreness of the quadriceps femoris. *Human Movement, 15*(4), pp. 234–237.

Brooks, C.P., Woodruff, L.D., Wright, L.L. and Donatelli, R., 2005. The immediate effects of manual massage on power-grip performance after maximal exercise in healthy adults. *Journal of Alternative & Complementary Medicine: Research on Paradigm, Practice, and Policy, 11*(6), pp. 1093–1101.

Caldwell, E., 2001. *Remedial massage therapy.* Fishbourne, Chichester: Corpus Publishing Limited, pp. 35–41.

Cè, E., Limonta, E., Maggioni, M.A., Rampichini, S., Veicsteinas, A. and Esposito, F., 2013. Stretching and deep and superficial massage do not influence blood lactate levels after heavy-intensity cycle exercise. *Journal of Sports Sciences, 31*(8), pp. 856–866.

Cheung, K., Hume, P.A. and Maxwell, L., 2003. Delayed onset muscle soreness. *Sports Medicine, 33*(2), pp. 145–164.

Connolly, D.A., Sayers, S.P. and McHugh, M.P., 2003. Treatment and prevention of delayed onset muscle soreness. *Journal of Strength and Conditioning Research, 17*(1), pp. 197–208.

Crane, J.D., Ogborn, D.I., Cupido, C., Melov, S., Hubbard, A., Bourgeois, J.M. and Tarnopolsky, M.A., 2012. Massage therapy attenuates inflammatory signaling after exercise-induced muscle damage. *Science Translational Medicine, 4*(119), pp. 119ra13–119ra13.

Dariusz, B., Sylwia, K., Grzegorz, A.J. and Dariusz, B., 2014. Assessment of effectiveness of sports massage in supporting of warm-up. *Pedagogy of Physical Culture and Sports,* (10).

Davis, H.L., Alabed, S. and Chico, T.J.A., 2020. Effect of sports massage on performance and recovery: A systematic review and meta-analysis. *BMJ Open Sport & Exercise Medicine, 6*(1), p. e000614.

Dawson, L.G., Dawson, K.A. and Tiidus, P.M., 2004. Evaluating the influence of massage on leg strength, swelling, and pain following a half-marathon. *Journal of Sports Science & Medicine, 3*(YISI 1), p. 37.

Delextrat, A., Calleja-González, J., Hippocrate, A. and Clarke, N.D., 2013. Effects of sports massage and intermittent cold-water immersion on recovery from matches by basketball players. *Journal of Sports Sciences, 31*(1), pp. 11–19.

Drust, B., Atkinson, G., Gregson, W., French, D. and Binningsley, D., 2003. The effects of massage on intra-muscular temperature in the vastus lateralis in humans. *International Journal of Sports Medicine, 24*(06), pp. 395–399.

Duñabeitia, I., Arrieta, H., Rodriguez-Larrad, A., Gil, J., Esain, I., Gil, S.M., Irazusta, J. and Bidaurrazaga-Letona, I., 2019. Effects of massage and cold-water immersion after an exhaustive run on running economy and biomechanics: A Randomized Controlled Trial. *Journal of Strength and Conditioning Research.* doi: 10.1519/jsc.0000000000003395

Dupuy, O., Douzi, W., Theurot, D., Bosquet, L. and Dugué, B., 2018. An evidence-based approach for choosing post-exercise recovery techniques to reduce markers of muscle damage, soreness, fatigue, and inflammation: a systematic review with meta-analysis. *Frontiers in Physiology, 9*, p. 403.

Eriksson Crommert, M., Lacourpaille, L., Heales, L.J., Tucker, K. and Hug, F., 2015. Massage induces an immediate, albeit short-term, reduction in muscle stiffness. *Scandinavian Journal of Medicine & Science in Sports, 25*(5), pp. e490–e496.

Farr, T., Nottle, C., Nosaka, K. and Sacco, P., 2002. The effects of therapeutic massage on delayed onset muscle soreness and muscle function following downhill walking. *Journal of Science and Medicine in Sport, 5*(4), pp. 297–306.

Field, T., Hernandez-Reif, M., Diego, M., Schanberg, S. and Kuhn, C., 2005. Cortisol decreases and serotonin and dopamine increase following massage therapy. *International Journal of Neuroscience*, 115(10), pp. 1397–1413.

Fletcher, I.M., 2010. The effects of precompetition massage on the kinematic parameters of 20-m sprint performance. *The Journal of Strength & Conditioning Research*, 24(5), pp. 1179–1183.

Goodwin, J.E., Glaister, M., Howatson, G., Lockey, R.A. and McInnes, G., 2007. Effect of preperformance lower-limb massage on thirty-meter sprint running. *Journal of Strength and Conditioning Research*, 21(4), p. 1028.

Guo, J., Li, L., Gong, Y., Zhu, R., Xu, J., Zou, J. and Chen, X., 2017. Massage alleviates delayed onset muscle soreness after strenuous exercise: A systematic review and meta-analysis. *Frontiers in physiology*, 8, p. 747.

Hall, J.E., 2010. *Guyton and Hall textbook of medical physiology: Enhanced E-book*. Philadelphia, PA: Elsevier Health Sciences.

Hart, J.M., Swanik, C.B. and Tierney, R.T., 2005. Effects of sport massage on limb girth and discomfort associated with eccentric exercise. *Journal of Athletic Training*, 40(3), p. 181.

Hemmings, B., Smith, M., Graydon, J. and Dyson, R., 2000. Effects of massage on physiological restoration, perceived recovery, and repeated sports performance. *British Journal of Sports Medicine*, 34(2), pp. 109–114.

Hinds, T., McEwan, I., Perkes, J., Dawson, E., Ball, D. and George, K. 2004. Effects of massage on limb and skin blood flow after quadriceps exercise. *Medicine & Science in Sports & Exercise*, 195(9131/04), pp. 3608–1308.

Holub, C. and Smith, J.D., 2017. Effect of Swedish massage on DOMS after strenuous exercise. *International Journal of Exercise Science*, 10(2), pp. 258–265.

Hopper, D., Deacon, S., Das, S., Jain, A., Riddell, D., Hall, T. and Briffa, K., 2005. Dynamic soft tissue mobilisation increases hamstring flexibility in healthy male subjects. *British Journal of Sports Medicine*, 39(9), pp. 594–598.

Howatson, G. and Van Someren, K.A., 2008. The prevention and treatment of exercise-induced muscle damage. *Sports Medicine*, 38(6), pp. 483–503.

Huang, S.Y., Di Santo, M., Wadden, K.P., Cappa, D.F., Alkanani, T. and Behm, D.G., 2010. Short-duration massage at the hamstrings musculotendinous junction induces greater range of motion. *The Journal of Strength & Conditioning Research*, 24(7), pp. 1917–1924.

Hunter, A.M., Watt, J.M., Watt, V. and Galloway, S.D.R., 2006. Effect of lower limb massage on electromyography and force production of the knee extensors. *British Journal of Sports Medicine*, 40(2), pp. 114–118.

Imtiyaz, S., Veqar, Z. and Shareef, M.Y., 2014. To compare the effect of vibration therapy and massage in prevention of delayed onset muscle soreness (DOMS). *Journal of Clinical and Diagnostic Research: JCDR*, 8(1), p. 133.

Jooste, K., Khumalo, V. and Maritz, J., 2013. Sportmen's experiences at a somatology clinic receiving a sport massage. *Health SA Gesondheid (Online)*, 18(1), pp. 1–9.

Kalman, D., Knight, K., Sperry, J., Smith, M. and Holms, C., 2018. A randomized double-blind placebo controlled clinical trial evaluating the effects of an investigational study product on exercise induced muscle soreness, markers of inflammation, muscle damage and exercise performance in healthy males. *Journal of Nutrition and Health Sciences*, 5(1), p. 104.

Kargarfard, M., Lam, E.T., Shariat, A., Shaw, I., Shaw, B.S. and Tamrin, S.B., 2016. Efficacy of massage on muscle soreness, perceived recovery, physiological restoration and physical performance in male bodybuilders. *Journal of Sports Sciences*, 34(10), pp. 959–965.

Kaur, K. and Sinha, A.G.K., 2020. Effectiveness of massage on flexibility of hamstring muscle and agility of female players: an experimental randomized controlled trial. *Journal of Bodywork and Movement Therapies*, 24(4), pp. 519–526.

Kennedy, A.B., Patil, N. and Trilk, J.L., 2018. 'Recover quicker, train harder, and increase flexibility': massage therapy for elite para-cyclists, a mixed-methods study. *BMJ Open Sport & Exercise Medicine*, 4(1), p. e000319. doi:10.1136/bmjsem-2017-000319

Khamwong, P., Pirunsan, U. and Paungmali, A., 2010. The prophylactic effect of massage on symptoms of muscle damage induced by eccentric exercise of the wrist extensors. *Journal of Sports Science and Technology*, 10(1), p. 245.

Laux, P., Krumm, B., Diers, M. and Flor, H., 2015. Recovery–stress balance and injury risk in professional football players: a prospective study. *Journal of Sports Sciences*, 33(20), pp. 2140–2148.

Law, L.A.F., Evans, S., Knudtson, J., Nus, S., Scholl, K. and Sluka, K.A., 2008. Massage reduces pain perception and hyperalgesia in experimental muscle pain: A randomized, controlled trial. *The Journal of Pain*, 9(8), pp. 714–721.

Leivadi, S., Hernandez-Reif, M., Field, T., O'Rourke, M., D'Arienzo, S., Lewis, D., Pino, N.D., Schanberg, S. and Kuhn, C., 1999. Massage therapy and relaxation effects on university dance students. *Journal of Dance Medicine & Science*, 3(3), pp. 108–112.

Lewis, P.B., Ruby, D. and Bush-Joseph, C.A., 2012. Muscle soreness and delayed-onset muscle soreness. *Clinics in Sports Medicine*, 31(2), pp. 255–262.

MacIntyre, D.L., Sorichter, S., Mair, J., Berg, A. and McKenzie, D.C., 2001. Markers of inflammation and myofibrillar proteins following eccentric exercise in humans. *European Journal of Applied Physiology*, 84(3), pp. 180–186.

Mancinelli, C.A., Davis, D.S., Aboulhosn, L., Brady, M., Eisenhofer, J. and Foutty, S., 2006. The effects of massage on delayed onset muscle soreness and physical performance in female collegiate athletes. *Physical Therapy in Sport*, 7(1), pp. 5–13.

McKechnie, G.J., Young, W.B. and Behm, D.G., 2007. Acute effects of two massage techniques on ankle joint flexibility and power of the plantar flexors. *Journal of Sports Science & Medicine*, 6(4), p. 498.

Micklewright, D., Griffin, M., Gladwell, V. and Beneke, R., 2005. Mood state response to massage and subsequent exercise performance. *The Sport Psychologist*, 19(3), pp. 234–250.

Micklewright, D., Sellens, M., Gladwell, V. and Beneke, R., 2006. Blood lactate removal using combined massage and active recovery. *Biology of Sport*, 23(4), p. 315.

Molouki, A., Hosseini, S.M., Rustaee, M. and Tabatabaee, S.M., 2016. The immediate effects of manual massage of forearm on power-grip strength and endurance in healthy young men. *Journal of Chiropractic Medicine*, 15(2), pp. 112–120.

Moran, R.N., Hauth, J.M. and Rabena, R., 2018. The effect of massage on acceleration and sprint performance in track & field athletes. *Complementary Therapies in Clinical Practice*, 30, pp. 1–5.

Morasaka A. 2005. Sports massage a comprehensive review. *Journal of Sports Medicine and Physical Fitness*, 45, pp. 370–380.

Mori, H., Ohsawa, H., Tanaka, T.H., Taniwaki, E., Leisman, G. and Nishijo, K., 2004. Effect of massage on blood flow and muscle fatigue following isometric lumbar exercise. *Medical Science Monitor*, 10(5), pp. CR173–CR178.

Mostafaloo, A., 2012. The effect of one session massage in the lower limb muscle on flexibility, power and agility tests performance in soccer players. *Journal of Jahrom University of Medical Sciences*, 10(2), p. 19.

Moyer, C.A., Seefeldt, L., Mann, E.S. and Jackley, L.M., 2011. Does massage therapy reduce cortisol? A comprehensive quantitative review. *Journal of Bodywork and Movement Therapies*, 15(1), pp. 3–14.

Noto, Y., Kudo, M. and Hirota, K., 2010. Back massage therapy promotes psychological relaxation and an increase in salivary chromogranin A release. *Journal of Anesthesia*, 24(6), pp. 955–958.

Ntshangase, S. and Peters-Futre, E., 2017. The efficacy of manual versus local vibratory massage in promoting recovery from post-exercise muscle damage–A systematic review. *Journal of Science and Medicine in Sport*, 20, p. e42.

Nunes, G.S., Bender, P.U., de Menezes, F.S., Yamashitafuji, I., Vargas, V.Z. and Wageck, B., 2016. Massage therapy decreases pain and perceived fatigue after long-distance Ironman triathlon: a randomised trial. *Journal of Physiotherapy*, 62(2), pp. 83–87.

Paine T., 2000. *The complete guide to sports massage* (Vol. 9, pp. 79–114). London: A & C Black Publishing Ltd.

Pinar, S., Kaya, F., Bicer, B., Erzeybek, M.S. and Cotuk, H.B., 2012. Different recovery methods and muscle performance after exhausting exercise: Comparison of the effects of electrical muscle stimulation and massage. *Biology of Sport*, 29(4), p. 269.

Pinar, R. and Afsar, F., 2016. Back massage to decrease state anxiety, cortisol level, blood pressure, heart rate and increase sleep quality in family caregivers of patients with cancer: A randomised controlled trial. *Asian Pacific Journal of Cancer Prevention*, 16(18), pp. 8127–8133.

Rasooli, S.A., Jahromi, M.K., Asadmanesh, A. and Salesi, M., 2012. Influence of massage, active and passive recovery on swimming performance and blood lactate. *Journal of Sport Medicine and Physical Fitness*, 52, pp. 122–127.

Romadhona, N.F., Sari, G.M. and Utomo, D.N., 2019. Comparison of sport massage and combination of cold-water immersion with sport massage on decrease of blood lactic acid level. In *IOP Conference Series: Journal of Physics* (No. 1146, pp. 01–04). IOP Publishing Ltd.

Sarli, D. and Agus, M., 2014. Research articles the effect of differences oxytocin levels through oxytocin massage against number of bleeding in mother 2 hours postpartum. *Jurnal Kesehatan Andalas*, 4(3), pp. 743–750.

Sefton, J.M., Yarar, C., Berry, J.W. and Pascoe, D.D., 2010. Therapeutic massage of the neck and shoulders produces changes in peripheral blood flow when assessed with dynamic infrared thermography. *The Journal of Alternative and Complementary Medicine*, 16(7), pp. 723–732.

Shah, Y., Arkesteijn, M., Thomas, D., Whyman, J. and Passfield, L., 2017. The acute effects of integrated myofascial techniques on lumbar paraspinal blood flow compared with kinesio-taping: A pilot study. *Journal of Bodywork and Movement Therapies*, 21(2), pp. 459–467.

Shin, M.S. and Sung, Y.H., 2015. Effects of massage on muscular strength and proprioception after exercise-induced muscle damage. *The Journal of Strength & Conditioning Research*, 29(8), pp. 2255–2260.

Szabo, A., Rendi, M., Szabó, T., Velenczei, A. and Kovács, Á., 2008. Psychological effects of massage on running. *Journal of Social, Behavioral, and Health Sciences*, 2(1), p. 1.

Veqar, Z. and Kalra, R., 2013. Causes and management of delayed onset muscle soreness: A review. *Elixir Human Physio*, 55, pp. 13205–11.

Visconti, L., Capra, G., Carta, G., Forni, C. and Janin, D., 2015. Effect of massage on DOMS in ultramarathon runners: A pilot study. *Journal of Bodywork and Movement Therapies*, 19(3), pp. 458–463.

Visconti, L., Forni, C., Coser, R., Trucco, M., Magnano, E. and Capra, G., 2020. Comparison of the effectiveness of manual massage, long-wave diathermy, and sham long-wave diathermy for the management of delayed-onset muscle soreness: A randomized controlled trial. *Archives of Physiotherapy*, 10(1), pp. 1–7.

Weerapong, P., Hume, P.A. and Kolt, G.S., 2005. The mechanisms of massage and effects on performance, muscle recovery and injury prevention. *Sports Medicine*, 35(3), pp. 235–256.

Wiltshire, E.V., Poitras, V., Pak, M., Hong, T., Rayner, J. and Tschakovsky, M.E., 2010. Massage impairs postexercise muscle blood flow and 'lactic acid' removal. *Medicine & Science in Sports & Exercise*, 42(6), pp. 1062–1071.

Yeun, Y.R., 2017. Effectiveness of massage therapy on the range of motion of the shoulder: A systematic review and meta-analysis. *Journal of Physical Therapy Science*, 29(2), pp. 365–369.

Zadkhosh, S.M., Ariaee, E., Atri, A., Rashidlamir, A. and Saadatyar, A., 2015. The effect of massage therapy on depression, anxiety and stress in adolescent wrestlers. *International Journal of Sport Studies*, 5(3), pp. 321–327.

Zainuddin, Z., Newton, M., Sacco, P. and Nosaka, K., 2005. Effects of massage on delayed-onset muscle soreness, swelling, and recovery of muscle function. *Journal of Athletic Training*, 40(3), p. 174.

Zusman, M., 2013. Belief reinforcement: one reason why costs for low back pain have not decreased. *Journal of Multidisciplinary Healthcare*, 6, p. 197.

7 Stretching

Stretch Reflexes

The Golgi tendon organ (GTO) provides a signal related to the tension of tendons and is commonly found in the muscle-tendon complex (MTC) near the origin and insertion. GTOs are classically seen and empirically proven to signal tendon force; however, Kistemaker et al. (2013) argued that simply because tendon length is dependent on tendon force, GTOs can just as well be seen (and proven) to signal tendon length. As such, spindle and GTOs together should be able to sense MTC length. The stretch reflex or myotatic reflex refers to the contraction of a muscle in response to its passive stretching by increasing its contractility, as long as the stretch is within physiological limits. When a muscle lengthens, the muscle spindle located inside the muscle is stretched, and the rate of neural firing of muscle spindle afferents increases (Bhattacharyya, 2017). Anatomical and physiological analyses have long revealed differences between proprioceptive groups Ia/II and Ib sensory neurons, yet the molecular correlates of these three muscle afferent subtypes remain unknown. Oliver et al. (2020) performed single-cell RNA sequencing of genetically identified adult proprioceptors and, using unbiased bioinformatics approaches, detected five molecularly distinct neuronal clusters. Validation of cluster-specific transcripts in dorsal root ganglia (DRG) and skeletal muscle provides evidence that these clusters correspond to functionally distinct muscle spindle (MS) or GTO afferent proprioceptors. Remarkably, the authors uncovered just one type of GTO afferent, while four of the five clusters represent MS afferents, thus demonstrating a previously unappreciated diversity among these muscle proprioceptors. This diversity in muscle proprioceptors highlights why individual athletes may demonstrate different physiological outcomes to stretching protocols.

Static and Dynamic Stretching

- Static stretching – a muscle is held in a position of minimal discomfort for a period of time, usually between 10 and 30 seconds.
- Dynamic stretching – constant movement of a muscle into an extended range of motion, not exceeding the athlete's static-passive stretching ability.

Although it is beyond the scope of this book to fully explore the science and practice of stretching for improved sports performance outcomes, it is considered the most therapeutic technique to improve and maintain muscle length (Nagarwal et al., 2010). However, it has been noted (Behm et al., 2016) that both static stretching and proprioceptive neuromuscular facilitation (PNF) stretching show no overall effect on all-cause injury or overuse injuries, but there may be a benefit in reducing acute muscle injuries with running, sprinting or other repetitive

DOI: 10.4324/9781003104803-7

contractions. Changes may result from acute reductions in muscle and tendon stiffness or from neural adaptations causing an improved stretch tolerance. Results from a study by Avloniti and co-workers (2016) suggested that a short-duration static stretch (SS) protocol induced acute improvements in speed and agility performance, whereas longer-duration SS protocols had neither a positive nor a negative effect. Furthermore, it seems that individuals of lower speed and agility performance levels are more likely to benefit from a short-duration SS protocol.

Static stretching prior to performance still remains controversial, with some studies reporting negative effects on sprinting (Nelson et al., 2005; Fletcher & Anness, 2007) and jump performance (not sprint time) (Vetter, 2007; Pearce et al., 2009) due to a decrease in the muscle-tendon unit's (MTU) ability to store and release elastic energy (Fletcher & Anness, 2007). However, others disagree; for example, Samson et al.'s, study (2012) on the effects of static and dynamic stretching protocols within general and activity-specific warm ups noted no differences in sprint performance (6 × 20 m) between dynamic and static stretch groups in the absence of a sport-specific warm up. The static stretch condition increased sit and reach range of motion (ROM) by 2.8% more ($p = 0.0083$) than the dynamic condition.

Contrary to this, Opplert and Babault (2018) found dynamic stretching represents a more efficient modality than static stretching when employed prior to subsequent muscular performance, and especially prior to explosive or high-speed activities. In agreement, Lin et al. (2020) suggested practitioners should consider dynamic stretching as a first line of warm-up exercise to increase ROM, CMJ height, and agility in athletes. However, it would appear that with static stretching, the longer the static stretch is held, the more likely it could have a detrimental effect on subsequent performance. This point was highlighted in Behm and Chaouachi's extensive review in 2011. The authors identified a duration of greater than 90 seconds of static stretching as a common duration in the literature where static stretching generally produced impairments. Wong et al. (2011) also noted 30-, 60- and 90-second stretches had no detrimental effect on repeated sprint ability or change of direction speed. The authors suggested the short duration (≤ 90 s) static stretching may not have provided sufficient stimulus to elicit performance impairments. This concurs with a study by Stafilidis and Tilp (2015), who also noted that an applied stretch stimuli (15 or 60 seconds) was not sufficient to trigger adaptations in the mechano-morphological properties of the lower extremities' MTUs, which therefore affected neither jump performance nor maximal voluntary contraction (MVC) when static (passive) or dynamic stretching were incorporated into a warm-up routine. Blazevich et al. (2018) highlighted that, after a low-intensity warm up, which consisted of a 3-minute jog, 5 seconds of high knees and 5 seconds of heel to butt, a 5-second static stretch (5S), 30-second static stretch (30S; 3 × 10-second stretches), five-repetition (per muscle group) dynamic stretch (DYN), or no stretch (NS), was performed. The authors results found no effects on sprint running, jumping or change of direction compared to no stretching. However, the authors speculated that it allowed for individuals to feel more confident of high performance in the ensuing sports-related tests, indicating there was a psychological effect. Hence, they concluded, both short or moderate-duration static stretching should be allowed prior to exercise.

In an acute setting, Santos et al. (2020) investigated the effects of different stretching intensities on the range of motion (ROM), passive torque and muscle architecture. The authors concluded both high or low intensity stretching acutely promotes similar gains in flexibility, that is, there are short-term/immediate gains in ROM, but it does not modify passive torque and muscle architecture. In addition, following a 3 × 60-second stretching exercise, Konrad and Tilp (2020) found an increase in range of motion, a decrease in peak relative torque and a decrease in muscle stiffness, both immediately and 5 minutes after stretching, with no changes detected in maximal voluntary contraction at any time. Furthermore, the authors found no effect on tendon tissue properties at any time following the stretching. With this in mind, short-duration stretches of high or low intensity are unlikely to be detrimental to athletic performance and may increase range of motion, and offer some psychological reassurance to the athlete.

Assisted Stretching

When stretching an athlete it is important to have the limb fully supported, enabling the athlete to fully relax the muscle being stretched. It may be necessary to stabilise other joints to minimise compensatory movements. The therapist should obtain regular feedback to measure the intensity of the stretch, aiming for minimal discomfort levels rather than pain towards the end of the range. This type of assisted static stretch is typically held for approximately 30–60 seconds and can be repeated 2–3 times per limb.

Assisted stretching examples are shown in Figures 7.1a, 7.1b and 7.1c.

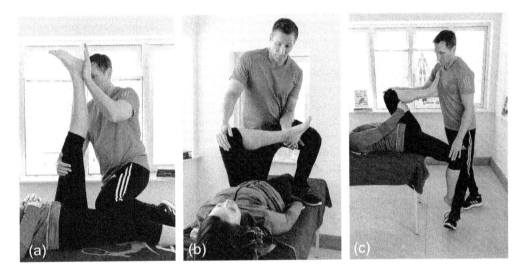

Figure 7.1 (a) Hamstrings. (b) Gluteals. (c) Hip flexors.

Advanced Techniques

Muscle Energy Technique (MET)

METs are used by therapists to increase muscle extensibility (visco-elastic properties), decrease muscle hyper-tonicity and improve joint range of motion, through the influence of the Golgi tendon. This type of assisted stretching includes post-isometric relaxation (PIR), reciprocal inhibition (RI) and contract-relax (CR) stretching. MET uses the voluntary contraction of the patient's muscle in a precisely controlled direction against an externally applied counterforce, which is applied by the operator (Franke et al., 2015). The mechanisms behind the use of MET still remains unclear, but it is likely to be largely neurological and induces hypoalgesia and altered proprioception.

In a study by Patel et al. (2018) comparisons were drawn between MET and MET-SCS (strain-counterstrain) groups. The authors found both to be equal in terms of a reduction of low back pain and disability, although after the second day of treatment adding SCS did not provide any greater results than MET alone. Equally, Kannabiran (2015) concluded there was no difference in low back pain (using VAS) or range of motion when comparing MET with positional release techniques, with both groups providing good results in the management of mechanical low back pain. Furthermore, in a study by Fahrmy et al (2019), patients received muscle energy technique involving isometric contraction of the agonist muscle for 10 seconds, with the contraction starting just short of the restricted range. After that, the patient was asked to relax for 2–3 seconds, then the examiner stretched the contracted muscle in the opposite direction for 10 seconds. This was repeated for three repetitions for each muscle bilaterally. The authors' results indicated that muscle energy technique was better than extension exercises for decreasing pain and functional disability in patients with chronic mechanical low back pain, but the extension exercise program had a better effect on improving lumbar range of motion.

Jalal et al. (2018) treated patients using muscle energy technique for cervical pain and range of motion. Results showed clinically an improvement in a number of different range of motions, including cervical flexion, cervical extension, cervical right-side rotation ($p = 0.001$), cervical left side rotation cervical right side bending and cervical left side bending ($p = 0.01$), and in subjective pain levels (VAS). Additionally, Jeong et al. (2017) demonstrated that passive stretching massage and MET (2 sets of 3 10-second repetitions of isometric resistance exercise, followed by 10 seconds of rest) are effective methods for improving ROM, strength and pressure pain threshold (PPT) for musculoskeletal neck pain.

Muscle energy technique, proprioceptive neuromuscular facilitation technique and a self-stretching control group were compared in subjects with chronic mechanical neck pain by Kumari et al. (2016). The authors found statistically significant improvement ($p < 0.05$) in all the three groups, with MET and PNF groups equally effective. These results are likely to come from a reduction in muscle spasm, or tightness reflex relaxation and viscoelastic changes, by first resetting the muscle spindle and inhibiting the muscles by activating the Golgi tendon. Other studies have concluded that MET is an effective treatment for increasing the ROM and strength of internal rotation at the glenohumeral joint in asymptomatic overhead athletes (Sehgal et al., 2016). In addition, Contractor et al. (2016) discovered that METs are more effective than conventional treatment in increasing range of motion in patients with adhesive capsulitis (conventional treatment included short wave diathermy [SWD], 20 minutes with capacitor field method, Codman's exercises, rope and pulley, wall and ladder exercise, shoulder wheel exercise, self-stretching exercise). Therefore, METs have demonstrated positive results in the upper and lower body and could be a useful option when trying to increase an athlete's range of motion. On a negative note, a Cochrane database of systematic reviews conducted by Franke et al. (2015) concluded that the quality of research related to testing the effectiveness of MET is poor. The authors stated that studies are generally small and have a high risk of bias due to methodological deficiencies.

Post Iso-Metrical Relaxation (PIR)

In PIR, the target muscle is contracted using autogenic inhibition (GTOs override the muscle spindles which facilitates relaxation and reduced tension in the muscle).

Redij et al. (2017) compared PIR and MET in order to improve flexibility in the iliopsoas muscle in 30 male and female students. The techniques were performed three times for three weeks. The authors' results indicated a significant improvement in iliopsoas flexibility in both MET and PIR groups, with the MET group having a greater improvement than the PIR group (t = 3.198, p < 0.0001). In another study (Agrawal, 2016), this time comparing PIR against reciprocal inhibition (RI) on hamstring length (n = 100), both groups demonstrated improvements in hamstring flexibility (p = 0.000), but the PIR group showed greater improvement than the RI group (p = 0.000). Other studies have also noted improvements in hamstring range of motion and flexibility using PIR techniques (Islam et al., 2017), and with a combination of cross frictional massage on ankle joint dorsiflexion (Yadav et al., 2016).

Reciprocal Inhibition (RI)/Contract-Relax (CR)

With the limb fully supported, the athlete uses approximately 25–50% of their muscular strength to push against the therapist (isometric contraction) for 4 ×10-second stretches plus 5-second contractions (Kay et al., 2016). Other durations of stretch and contraction have also been used in the literature, for example 5 × 7-second stretches plus 7-second contractions (Spernoga et al., 2001; Ahmed et al., 2015).

A number of articles have demonstrated improvements in range of motion using contract-relax stretching and static stretching (Feland et al., 2001; Lim et al., 2014; Ahmed et al., 2015). These improvements could be as a result of stretch tolerance or as a result of autogenic inhibition. However, Yavuz et al.'s 2018 research highlighted the difficulty when comparisons are made between muscle groups. The authors demonstrated that the strength of reciprocal inhibition in the tibialis anterior motor units was fourfold greater than for the gastrocnemius muscle and the soleus motor units. The authors suggested this asymmetry cannot be explained by differences in motor unit type composition between the investigated muscles, as they sampled low-threshold motor units in all cases. Therefore, the differences observed for the strength of inhibition was presumably due to a differential reciprocal spindle afferent input and the relative contribution of nonreciprocal inhibitory pathways.

In a study by Burgess et al. (2019) on contract-relax-agonist-contract (CRAC) stretching, the antagonists (the hamstrings) were first passively stretched for 15 seconds, followed by a 6-second isometric contraction against resistance at the point of limitation. This contraction was immediately followed by a 6-second concentric contraction of the agonists (the quadriceps) followed by 20 seconds of rest, before the cycle was repeated three times. The authors demonstrated an increase in range of motion of 37% without any effect on agility or sprint times. This has an implication in sports where an increased range of motion is required without a detrimental effect on subsequent performance.

To summarise, an isometric contraction of a stretched muscle triggers autogenic inhibition which stimulates the Golgi-tendon organs, and in a static stretch muscle relaxation takes place via the inverse myotatic stretch reflex. When the antagonist muscle contracts there is excitability of motor neurons causing reciprocal inhibition which allows the muscle to lengthen. However, in a field-based study by Kay et al. (2020) on non-partner contract-relax stretching (hamstrings), comparable increases in knee flexor ROM, reductions in stiffness and increases in stretch tolerance and elastic potential energy storage were observed after both contract-relax (CR) and stretch-return-contract (SRC) (non-partner) stretching, when performed in both laboratory (dynamometer) and field-based environments. The authors also noted, as no substantial activation of the α-motoneuron pool appeared to have occurred in any condition, that alterations in autogenic inhibition are also not likely to be an important mechanism underpinning the increases in ROM.

References

Agrawal, S.S., 2016. Comparison between post isometric relaxation and reciprocal inhibition manoeuvres on hamstring flexibility in young healthy adults: Randomized clinical trial. *International Journal of Medical Research & Health Sciences*, 5(1), pp. 33–37.

Ahmed, H., Iqbal, A., Anwer, S. and Alghadir, A., 2015. Effect of modified hold-relax stretching and static stretching on hamstring muscle flexibility. *Journal of Physical Therapy Science*, 27(2), pp. 535–538.

Avloniti, A., Chatzinikolaou, A., Fatouros, I.G., Avloniti, C., Protopapa, M., Draganidis, D., Stampoulis, T., Leontsini, D., Mavropalias, G., Gounelas, G. and Kambas, A., 2016. The acute effects of static stretching on speed and agility performance depend on stretch duration and conditioning level. *Journal of Strength and Conditioning Research*, 30(10), pp. 2767–2773.

Behm, D.G., Blazevich, A.J., Kay, A.D. and McHugh, M., 2016. Acute effects of muscle stretching on physical performance, range of motion, and injury incidence in healthy active individuals: A systematic review. *Applied Physiology, Nutrition, and Metabolism*, 41(1), pp. 1–11.

Behm, D.G. and Chaouachi, A., 2011. A review of the acute effects of static and dynamic stretching on performance. *European Journal of Applied Physiology*, 111(11), pp. 2633–2651.

Bhattacharyya, K.B., 2017. The stretch reflex and the contributions of C David Marsden. *Annals of Indian Academy of Neurology*, 20(1), p. 1.

Blazevich, A.J., Gill, N.D., Kvorning, T., Kay, A.D., Goh, A.G., Hilton, B., Drinkwater, E.J. and Behm, D.G., 2018. No effect of muscle stretching within a full, dynamic warm-up on athletic performance. *Medicine & Science in Sports & Exercise*, 50(6), pp. 1258–1266.

Burgess, T., Vadachalam, T., Buchholtz, K. and Jelsma, J., 2019. The effect of the contract-relax-agonist-contract (CRAC) stretch of hamstrings on range of motion, sprint and agility performance in moderately active males: A randomised control trial. *South African Journal of Sports Medicine*, 31(1), pp. 1–5.

Contractor, E.S., Agnihotri, D.S. and Patel, R.M., 2016. Effect of Muscle Energy Technique on Range of Motion in Cases of Patients with Adhesive Capsulitis. *International Journal of Health Sciences and Research (IJHSR)*, 6(9), pp. 252–256.

Fahmy, E., Shaker, H., Ragab, W., Helmy, H. and Gaber, M., 2019. Efficacy of spinal extension exercise program versus muscle energy technique in treatment of chronic mechanical low back pain. *The Egyptian Journal of Neurology, Psychiatry and Neurosurgery*, 55(1), pp. 1–6.

Feland, J.B., Myrer, J.W. and Merrill, R.M., 2001. Acute changes in hamstring flexibility: PNF versus static stretch in senior athletes. *Physical Therapy in Sport*, 2(4), pp. 186–193.

Fletcher, I.M. and Anness, R., 2007. The acute effects of combined static and dynamic stretch protocols on fifty-meter sprint performance in track-and-field athletes. *Journal of Strength and Conditioning Research*, 21(3), p. 784.

Franke, H., Fryer, G., Ostelo, R.W. and Kamper, S.J., 2015. Muscle energy technique for non-specific low-back pain. *Cochrane Database of Systematic Reviews*, (2), CD009852. doi: 10.1002/14651858.CD009852.pub2.

Islam, F., Arshad, K., Arif, M.A. and Bashir, M.S., 2017. Post isometric hamstring stretching; efficacy of post isometric hamstring stretching with and without cross frictional massage football. *Professional Medical Journal*, 24(8), pp. 1224–1231.

Jalal, Y., Ahmad, A., Rahman, A.U. and Daud, M., 2018. Effectiveness of muscle energy technique on cervical range of motion and pain. *JPMA. The Journal of the Pakistan Medical Association*, 68(5), pp. 811–813.

Jeong, H.M., Shim, J.H. and Suh, H.R., 2017. The passive stretching, massage, and muscle energy technique effects on range of motion, strength, and pressure pain threshold in musculoskeletal neck pain of young adults. *Physical Therapy Rehabilitation Science*, 6(4), pp. 196–201.

Kannabiran, B., 2015. A comparative study of the effectiveness of two manual therapy techniques on pain and lumbar range of motion in individuals with mechanical low back ache. *EC Orthopaedics*, 2, pp. 36–42.

Kay, A.D., Dods, S. and Blazevich, A.J., 2016. Acute effects of contract-relax (CR) stretch versus a modified CR technique. *European Journal of Applied Physiology*, 116(3), pp. 611–621.

Kay, A.D., Dixon, J., Bligh, L.D. and Blazevich, A.J., 2020. The external validity of a novel contract-relax stretching technique on knee flexor range of motion. *Scandinavian Journal of Medicine & Science in Sports*, 30(1), pp. 74–82.

Kistemaker, D.A., Van Soest, A.J.K., Wong, J.D., Kurtzer, I. and Gribble, P.L., 2013. Control of position and movement is simplified by combined muscle spindle and Golgi tendon organ feedback. *Journal of Neurophysiology*, 109(4), pp. 1126–1139.

Konrad, A. and Tilp, M., 2020. The time course of muscle-tendon unit function and structure following three minutes of static stretching. *Journal of Sports Science & Medicine*, 19(1), p. 52.

Kumari, C., Sarkar, B., Banerjee, D., Alam, S., Sharma, R. and Biswas, A., 2016. Efficacy of muscle energy technique as compared to proprioceptive neuromuscular facilitation technique in chronic mechanical neck pain: A randomized controlled trial. *International Journal of Health Sciences and Research*, 6, pp. 152–61.

Lim, K.I., Nam, H.C. and Jung, K.S., 2014. Effects on hamstring muscle extensibility, muscle activity, and balance of different stretching techniques. *Journal of Physical Therapy Science*, 26(2), pp. 209–213.

Lin, W.C., Lee, C.L. and Chang, N.J., 2020. Acute Effects of Dynamic Stretching Followed by Vibration Foam Rolling on Sports Performance of Badminton Athletes. *Journal of Sports Science & Medicine*, 19(2), p. 420.

Nagarwal, A.K., Zutshi, K., Ram, C.S., Zafar, R. and Hamdard, J., 2010. Improvement of hamstring flexibility: A comparison between two PNF stretching techniques. *International Journal of Sports Science and Engineering*, 4(1), pp. 25–33.

Nelson, A.G., Kokkonen, J. and Arnall, D.A., 2005. Acute muscle stretching inhibits muscle strength endurance performance. *The Journal of Strength & Conditioning Research*, 19(2), pp. 338–343.

Oliver, K.M., Florez-Paz, D.M., Badea, T.C., Mentis, G.Z., Menon, V. and de Nooij, J.C., 2020. Molecular development of muscle spindle and Golgi tendon organ sensory afferents revealed by single proprioceptor transcriptome analysis. *bioRxiv*.

Opplert, J. and Babault, N., 2018. Acute effects of dynamic stretching on muscle flexibility and performance: An analysis of the current literature. *Sports Medicine*, 48(2), pp. 299–325.

Patel, V.D., Eapen, C., Ceepee, Z. and Kamath, R., 2018. Effect of muscle energy technique with and without strain–counter-strain technique in acute low back pain—A randomized clinical trial. *Hong Kong Physiotherapy Journal*, 38(01), pp. 41–51.

Pearce, A.J., Kidgell, D.J., Zois, J. and Carlson, J.S., 2009. Effects of secondary warm up following stretching. *European Journal of Applied Physiology*, 105(2), pp. 175–183.

Redij, S.N., Rao, K., Raorane, N.S., Chaudhari, R.S., Gattani, S.S., Katariya, K.S. and Shingavi, S.S., 2017. Comparison of muscle energy technique and post isometric relaxation on Iliopsoas tightness to improve flexibility in healthy young individuals. *International Journal of Applied Research*, 3, pp. 16–21.

Samson, M., Button, D.C., Chaouachi, A. and Behm, D.G., 2012. Effects of dynamic and static stretching within general and activity specific warm-up protocols. *Journal of Sports Science & Medicine*, 11(2), p. 279.

Santos, C.X., Beltrão, N.B., Piraúa, A.L.T., Durigan, J.L.Q., Behm, D. and de Araújo, R.C., 2020. Static stretching intensity does not influence acute range of motion, passive torque, and muscle architecture. *Journal of Sport Rehabilitation*, 29(1), pp. 1–6.

Sehgal, S., Sen, S. and Dhawan, A., 2016. Effects of muscle energy technique in increasing range of motion and strength of glenohumeral internal rotator, in athletes with glenohumeral internal rotation deficit. *American Journal of Sports Science*, 4(2), pp. 43–48.

Spernoga, S.G., Uhl, T.L., Arnold, B.L. and Gansneder, B.M., 2001. Duration of maintained hamstring flexibility after a one-time, modified hold-relax stretching protocol. *Journal of Athletic Training*, 36(1), p. 44.

Stafilidis, S. and Tilp, M., 2015. Effects of short duration static stretching on jump performance, maximum voluntary contraction, and various mechanical and morphological parameters of the muscle–tendon unit of the lower extremities. *European Journal of Applied Physiology*, 115(3), pp. 607–617.

Vetter, R.E., 2007. Effects of six warm-up protocols on sprint and jump performance. *Journal of Strength and Conditioning Research, 21*(3), p. 819.

Wong, D.P., Chaouachi, A., Lau, P.W. and Behm, D.G., 2011. Short durations of static stretching when combined with dynamic stretching do not impair repeated sprints and agility. *Journal of Sports Science & Medicine, 10*(2), p. 408.

Yadav N, Joshi S, Punia S. 2016. Immediate effect of soleus trigger point pressure release and post isometric relaxation (MET) on restricted active ankle joint dorsi-flexion among college females. *International Journal of Physiotherapy and Research, 4*(3) pp. 1564–68.

Yavuz, U.Ş., Negro, F., Diedrichs, R. and Farina, D., 2018. Reciprocal inhibition between motor neurons of the tibialis anterior and triceps surae in humans. *Journal of Neurophysiology, 119*(5), pp. 1699–1706.

8 Common Injuries and Treatment Options

Achilles Tendinitis

Achilles tendinitis/tendinopathy is recognised by tenderness/pain in the Achilles area (shown in Figures 8.1 and 8.2 and Table 8.1), local swelling and impaired function. In the athletic population it is usually caused by large amounts of high-intensity or high-speed work or running on soft surfaces such as sand, all of which increases injury risk, with distance runners having a tenfold risk of developing Achilles tendinopathy (Maffulli et al., 2004). In addition, increased braking force and low surface stiffness are associated with increased risk of Achilles tendon injuries (Lorimer & Hume, 2016). Furthermore, tendon vascularity, gastrocnemius and soleus dysfunction, age, sex, body weight and height, pes cavus and lateral ankle instability are considered common intrinsic factors (Longo et al., 2018). Historically, pain associated with tendon overuse is referred to as tendinitis (Weinreb et al., 2014). As with other overuse

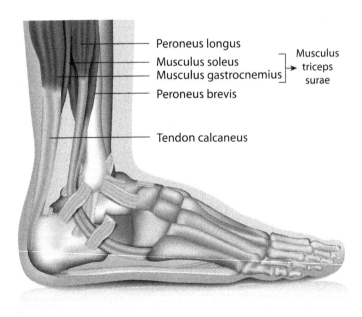

Figure 8.1 Triceps surae ankle joint (3D medical vector illustration).

DOI: 10.4324/9781003104803-8

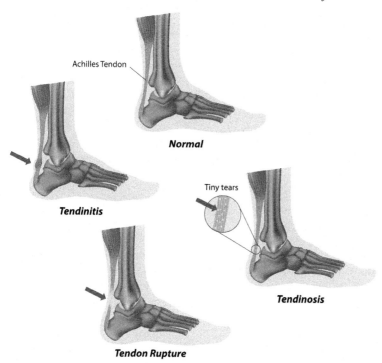

Figure 8.2 Achilles (calcaneal) tendon problems.

Table 8.1 Gastrocnemius and soleus

Muscle	Origin	Insertion	Action	Innervation
Gastrocnemius	Superior to articular surfaces of lateral condyle of femur and medial condyle of femur	Tendo-calcaneus into mid-posterior calcaneus	Plantar flexes foot, flexes knee	Tibial nerve, S1–S2
Soleus	Upper fibular, soleal line of tibia	Tendo-calcaneus	Plantar flexes the foot	Tibial nerve, L5–S2

related tendon injuries, inflammation at the site is not always found, but macroscopic changes including tendon thickening, loss of mechanical properties, and pain have been reported (Hodgson et al., 2012). During explosive activities such as jumping, a structurally and materially stiffer tendon enables an improved ability to transmit muscle-generated forces (Bojsen-Møller et al., 2005). A stiffer tendon that experiences less strain per unit force has a greater safety factor between functional and injurious tendon strains (Bayliss et al., 2016).

Over the past few years, the rate of surgically treated acute Achilles tendon ruptures has declined dramatically, with the argument continuing on whether surgical or non-surgical treatment is the best option. Still, there is no consensus over the ideal surgical procedure for the athletic population. If (percutaneous) surgery is selected, it has been reported that re-rupture rates are extremely low (2.1%) (Ververidis et al., 2016). However, it has been shown that athletes with a previous Achilles tendon rupture are 176 times more likely to suffer a contralateral Achilles tendon rupture compared to an individual without a previous rupture (Årøen et al., 2004). Additionally, athletes with weakened tendon integrity from repeated microtrauma during training combined with the sudden weight change distribution may be at risk of an Achilles tendon rupture. This devastating injury was shown to prevent return to play (RTP) for 30.6% of professional players (NBA, NFL, MBL) (Trofa et al., 2017) with successful return to play, game participation averaged 75.4% ($p = 0.001$) and 81.9% ($p = 0.002$) of the total games played the season before injury at one and two years postoperatively, respectively. This is likely to be a result of poor viscoelastic properties in the tendon, poor proprioception and weakness in the gastrocnemius-soleus complex.

To date, there is still no definitive or curative treatment for Achilles tendinopathy, but the use of deep friction massage still remains popular. Four hundred and seventy-eight physiotherapists completed an online questionnaire about their use of deep friction massage. Use of the technique was reported by 88.1% of the participants; tendinopathy was the clinical condition where it was most frequently used (84.9%) and within this 55.9% reported its use in degenerative tendinopathy (Chaves et al., 2017). The major Achilles tendon problems are shown in Figure 8.2.

Treatment Options for Achilles Tendinopathy

Following effleurage to warm the calf muscle area, continue with deeper work concentrating on the musculotendinous junction and the medial and lateral borders of the Achilles tendon (Figures 8.3a and 8.3b). Avoid direct pressure over the tendon itself. Petrissage, soft tissue release, deep circular frictions and trigger point therapy may be required to further relieve calf tightness. In chronic cases, cross fibre frictions and shockwave therapy should be considered. Isometric exercise from a suitably qualified health care professional, biomechanical advice, corrective footwear and training volume need to be investigated.

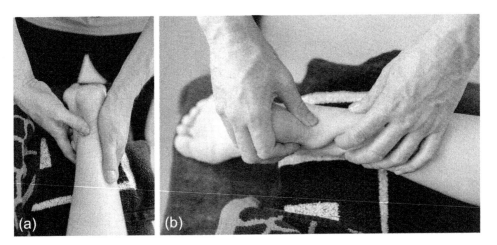

Figure 8.3 (a) Stabilise the foot using the thenar eminence of one hand whilst the thumb of the other pushes in a distal to proximal direction in small sections. (b) To mobilise the achilles tendon, use a gentle pincer grip to push and pull the tendon using the fingers on one hand, then the other, working through the length of the tendon.

Medial Tibial Stress Syndrome

The incidence of medial tibial stress syndrome (MTSS) has a reported rate ranging from 13.6% to 20% in runners (Lopes et al., 2012) and is generally accepted to be an overuse injury that causes pain at the onset of exercise felt along the posteromedial border of the tibia, usually in the middle or distal third of the bone; the anatomy of the area is shown in Figure 8.4 and Table 8.2. It occurs due to a combination of bone loading, biomechanical inefficiencies and

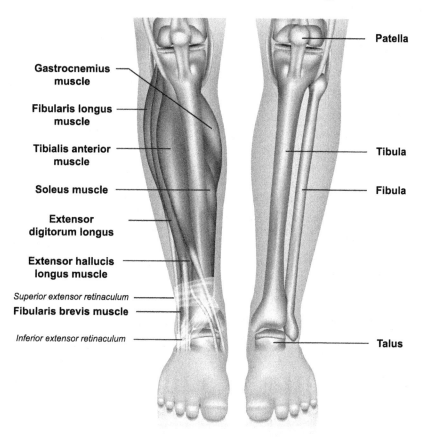

Figure 8.4 Lower leg anatomy.

Table 8.2 Tibialis posterior and flexor digitorum longus

Muscle	Origin	Insertion	Action	Innervation
Tibialis posterior	Tibia and fibula and interosseous membrane	Navicular and medial cuniform, bases of 2nd–4th metatarsals	Plantar flexion, foot inversion (supports medial longitudinal arch)	Tibial nerve, L4–L5
Flexor digitorum longus	Posterior surface of tibia	Plantar surface of bases of 2nd–5th distal phalanges	Inversion of foot, plantar flexes foot at ankle	Tibial nerve, L5, S1 and S2

myofascial traction and can be difficult to treat (McNamara et al., 2019). Metabolic events, vitamin deficiencies and decreased bone mineral density may also be the underlying causes (Ayan & Örsçelik, 2020). Initially the pain is experienced at the onset of activity and subsides with continued exercise, but later on the pain may persist even during activity (Moen et al., 2009).

Twenty-one studies were reviewed in a systematic review and meta-analysis by Hamstra-Wright et al. (2015). The authors determined that there were nine risk factors for developing MTSS, including individuals with increased BMI, navicular drop, plantar-flexion or hip external rotation, compared with their non-injured counterparts. It is also likely that traction on the periosteum and/or microtrauma of the musculature attaching onto the medial tibial border, tibialis posterior, flexor digitorum longus, soleus and deep crural fascia causes the pain experienced by athletes.

Treatment Options for MTSS (Shin Splints)

Following effleurage (superficial stroking) and petrissage to the gastrocnemius, tibialis posterior and soleus area, deeper work can begin. Deep stroking, circular fictions, ischemic compression (trigger points) and soft tissue release can all be used if they can be tolerated. Training footwear, biomechanical issues, running surface, training load and recovery need to be investigated.

When performing effleurage on the calf muscle (as shown in Figure 8.5), make sure a bolster or rolled towel is placed under the foot to relax the muscle. The therapist takes a long stance and keeps the back straight, with only a slight bend in the arms to minimise therapist fatigue. Working from above the musculotendinous junction, glide the hands along the limb finishing just below the knee. The hands then drag back to the start position. This can then be repeated 3–5 times as necessary.

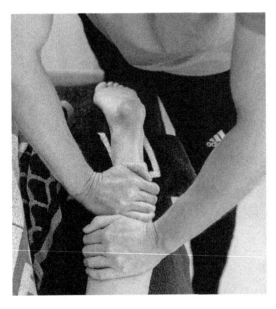

Figure 8.5 When performing effleurage on the calf muscle, make sure a bolster or rolled towel is placed under the foot to relax the muscle.

Petrissage is shown in Figures 8.6a and 8.6b. Both hands grasp the limb using the surface between the thumb and index finger. The hands then push towards the nearest lymph node 'cluster' (maintaining contact with the skin). The therapist then lifts (Figure 8.6b) and drags the hands back and then repeats this motion as many times as necessary.

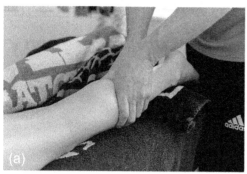
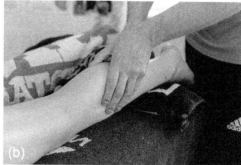

Figure 8.6 (a) Both hands grasp the limb using the surface between the thumb and index finger. (b) The therapist then lifts and drags the hands back and then repeats this motion as many times as necessary.

Figure 8.7 shows the therapist drawing the muscle away from the bone (away from the medial tibial border) to release the tension. Repeat as necessary.

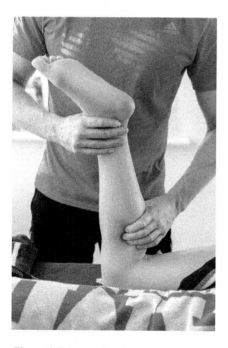

Figure 8.7 Draw the muscle away from the bone.

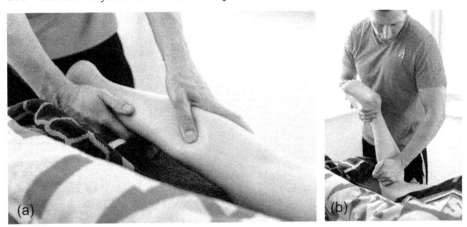

Figure 8.8 (a) Deeper stroking and circular frictions can be performed, using the thumb, or the heel of the hand. (b) Address tighter areas and adhesions.

Deeper stroking and circular frictions can be performed, using the thumb (Figure 8.8a) or the heel of the hand (Figure 8.8b) to address tighter areas and adhesions.

Anterior Knee Pain (Patellofemoral Pain Syndrome)

The anatomy of the knee is shown in Figure 8.9. Patellofemoral pain syndrome (PFPS) is a common orthopaedic problem that can cause serious disability, and it usually occurs due to chondromalacia patella (CMP). Injury to the patellar cartilage may develop as a result of patellofemoral morphological variations or anatomical incompatibility. This can lead to problems at the joint surface and an increase in the mechanical load on the normal joint surface (Aysin et al., 2018).

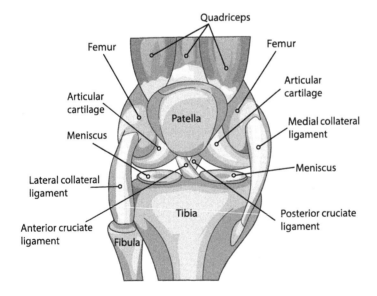

Figure 8.9 Knee joint cross section.

Anterior knee (patellofemoral) pain, is characterised by swelling and functional impairment in the anterior part of the knee, made worse by activity, prolonged sitting (with bent knees) and descending or ascending stairs. It is usually caused by overuse, poor training techniques and poor conditioning. The origin of pain could be in the lateral retinaculum, medial retinaculum, infrapatellar fat pad, synovium or the subchondral bone (Sanchis-Alfonso et al., 2020).

In athletically active men and women, the prevalence of anterior knee pain is reported to be 25% (Fredericson & Yoon, 2006). In addition, it has also been postulated that anterior knee pain is caused by malalignment and abnormal tracking of the patella, with vastus medialis oblique (see Table 8.3) playing an important role in stabilising the patella in the

Table 8.3 Vastus medialis oblique

Muscle	*Origin*	*Insertion*	*Actions*	*Innervation*
Vastus medialis oblique (part of the vastus medialis)	Medial side of femur (linear aspera)	Quadriceps tendon into tibial tubercle	Increases mechanical advantage of knee joint. Extends the knee, stabilises patella	Posterior division of femoral nerve L3–L4

femoral groove (Rothermich et al., 2015). However, although biomechanically appealing, the malalignment theory has failed to explain the presence of anterior knee pain in many patients, so other pathophysiologic processes must exist (Sanchis-Alfonso et al., 2020). Panken et al.'s 2015 systematic review of nine studies concluded with an interesting point. They stated that clinicians do not need to consider pain or activity-related pain for treatment decisions, as they appear to be unrelated to decreasing pain or increasing function in patients with anterior knee pain. At present, there is no consensus regarding the optimal treatment modality selection or expected time to recovery for anterior knee pain.

Special Tests

Clarke's Test

The athlete actively contracts the quadriceps muscle while the examiner's hand exerts pressure on the superior pole of the patella, trying to prevent the proximal movement of the patella. This test can reproduce discomfort. In normal subjects, however, reproduction of the symptoms does suggest pain of patellofemoral origin.

Patellofemoral Compression Test

The athlete sits on the table with the lower legs hanging over the side. The therapist compresses the patella while the athlete flexes and extends their leg within a 35-degree range. The flexion and extension can be done actively or passively. A positive test reproduces pain or discomfort, indicating patellofemoral syndrome.

Treatment Options for Anterior Knee Pain

After effleurage to the quadricep and iliotibial band area, use reinforced thumbs working distally to proximally up the length of the vastus lateralis, rectus femoris, tensor fascia lata, iliotibial band and into the gluteal muscles. Address any trigger points with ischemic compression. Other modalities including exercise therapy (gluteus medius and vastus medialis oblique strengthening), orthotics, ice, Kinesio-tape and dry needling (to trigger points) should also be considered.

Iliotibial Band Syndrome

The iliotibial band (ITB) is shown in Figure 8.10 and detailed further in Table 8.4. Iliotibial band syndrome (ITBS) occurs in 5% to 14% of runners; it is the leading cause of lateral knee pain and the second leading cause of overall knee pain in this population (Taunton et al., 2002; van der Worp et al., 2012). Previously, the condition was frequently referred to as iliotibial band friction syndrome. However, there is debate on whether iliotibial band syndrome is truly a friction syndrome, in which the ITB itself is pathologic, or whether a pathologic bursa forms

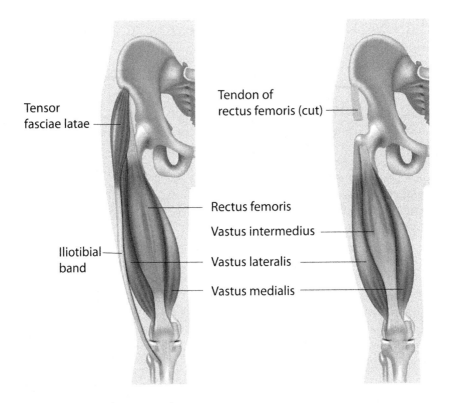

Figure 8.10 Quadriceps muscle.

Table 8.4 Iliotibial band

Muscle	Origin	Insertion	Action	Innervation
Iliotibial band (tract)	Anterolateral iliac tubercle portion of the external lip of the iliac crest	Lateral condyle of tibia (Gerdy's tubercle)	Extends, abducts and laterally rotates the hip. Contributes to lateral stabilisation of the knee	Superior gluteal nerve

between the ITB and the lateral femoral condyle, causing the pain (Beals & Flanigan, 2013). In a study by Antonio et al. (2013) the authors examined six cadavers and reported that the gluteus maximus presented a major insertion into the fascia lata, so large that the iliotibial tract could be considered a tendon of insertion of the gluteus maximus. The fascial insertion of the gluteus maximus muscle could explain the transmission of the forces from the thoracolumbar fascia to the knee. Taking this into account, therapists should treat the lower back, gluteal regions and fascia lata, rather than solely concentrating on the iliotibial band.

In a systematic review conducted by Louw & Deary (2014) involving distance runners, the authors noted those with a history of iliotibial band syndrome appear to have a number of biomechanical insufficiencies, including decreased rear foot eversion, internal tibial rotation, greater invertor moments at the feet and decreased abduction and flexion at the hips. In addition, on average male runners with ITBS have shown to have diminished ITB length (Noehren et al., 2014) which could exacerbate their symptoms, and could be an alternative explanation for iliotibial band syndrome. In cycling, the ITB is pulled anteriorly on the pedalling downstroke, and posteriorly on the upstroke. For those with an external tibia rotation of greater than 20 degrees, stress is created on the ITB if the athlete's cycling shoe is placed in a straight-ahead position or the toe is in a cleat position, and those with varus knee alignment or active pronation place a greater stretch on the distal ITB when they ride with internally rotated cleats (Nath, 2015). This could make potential irritation/inflammation more likely to occur as the iliotibial band slides over the lateral femoral condyle.

In a study of 16 asymptomatic individuals, Barton et al. (2014) found that both stretching alone and stretching combined with massage increased flexibility on the fascia lata complex by 3.4 degrees ($p < 0.01$) and 0.7 degrees ($p = 0.045$) respectively. However, whether this would have any long-term relief of symptoms is unclear. In addition, Friede et al. (2020) noted that following 6 weeks of physiotherapy, ITB stiffness actually increased by 14%, whilst pain and lower extremity function were significantly improved, leading the authors to suggest that current conservative management of ITBS appears to be ineffective at reducing ITB tone.

Traditionally, Ober's test and modified Ober's test (both described in the following section on special tests) have been used to assess ITB length. Findings by Willett et al. (2016) have refuted the hypothesis that the ITB plays a role in limiting hip adduction during either version of the Ober test, and questioned the validity of these tests for determining ITB tightness. However, it should be noted that the authors' study was performed on lightly embalmed cadavers.

Massage Techniques Around the Iliotibial Band and Tensor Fascia Lata

Make sure the athlete is in a comfortable position with towels positioned between the knees and ankles. Use one hand to support the limb as necessary whilst performing the technique, which is shown in Figures 8.11a, 8.11b and 8.11c. Use the thumb, palm or heel of the hand to massage the length of the iliotibial band through to the tensor fascia lata (without compressing the ITB onto the femur). Pay specific attention to the vastus lateralis and bicep femoris as they border the ITB. Excessive pressure during this technique is not necessary.

Special Tests

Obers Test

The athlete should be side-lying with the affected side uppermost. The bottom knee and hip should be flexed to flatten the lumbar curve. Standing behind the athlete, stabilise the pelvis/greater trochanter to prevent movement. Hold the distal end of the athlete's affected leg with

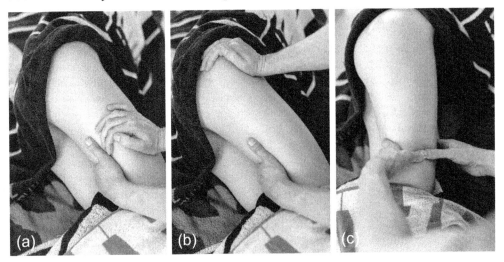

Figure 8.11 (a) Start. Work in small sections along the vastus lateralis, ITB and bicep femoris. (b) Finish. (c) Work distally to proximal in small sections.

your other hand and flex the leg to a right angle at the knee. Extend and abduct the hip joint and slowly lower the leg towards the massage couch – adduct the hip until motion is restricted. Make sure the hip does not internally rotate and flex during the test and the pelvis remains stabilised. If the thigh drops into flexion and internal rotation it will 'yield' to the tight tensor fascia lata and will not accurately test the length of the iliotibial band.

Modified Ober's Test

The athlete lies on their side with the underneath leg flexed at the hip and knee to flatten the lower back. The therapist stabilises the pelvis and keeps the lateral trunk in contact with the massage couch. A downward lateral tilt is equivalent to the hip abduction yielding to a tight tensor fascia lata. The therapist extends the leg, ensuring it is not internally rotated. If the leg fails to drop, a tight iliotibial band and tensor fascia lata is indicated – inter-rater reliability > 0.90 (Wang et al., 2006). It should be noted that Willett and colleagues (2016) refute the hypothesis that the ITB plays a role in limiting hip adduction during either version of the Ober test and question the validity of these tests for determining ITB tightness. The findings underscore the influence of the gluteus medius and minimus muscles as well as the hip joint capsule on Ober test findings.

Treatment Options for Iliotibial Band Syndrome

Following effleurage to warm the area, deep stroking techniques can be applied to the vastus lateralis, tensor fascia lata, bicep femoris and iliotibial band area. In a side-lying position used reinforced thumbs to get 'under' the ITB between its fascial attachments. Deep circular frictions and trigger pointing can be applied to the vastus lateralis, tensor fascia lata, gluteus medius and gluteus maximus. Biomechanical issues such as running technique and bike set-up need to be investigated, and gluteus medius strengthening exercises, training load, footwear and the use of appropriate recovery interventions all need to be addressed. Foam rolling can be used to apply ischemic compression to trigger points between massage sessions.

Lateral Epicondylitis (LE) – Tennis Elbow

The anatomy of the elbow is shown in Figure 8.12. Chronic pain in the common extensor at the origin of the lateral epicondyle, commonly called tennis elbow, is a condition with

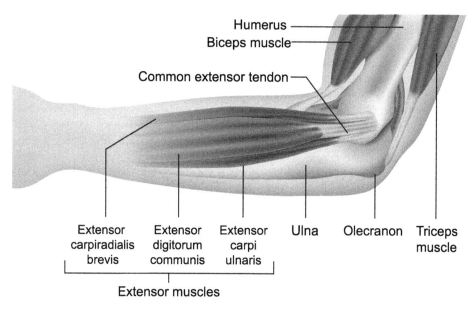

Figure 8.12 Anatomy of the elbow muscles (medical vector illustration).

unknown aetiology and pathogenesis (Ahmad et al., 2013; Luk et al., 2014). It is frequently caused by overuse or repetitive strain as a result of repeated extension (bending back) of the wrist against resistance, with the main pain generator related to the origin of the extensor carpi radialis brevis (ECRB) (outlined in Table 8.5), as a result of tendon compression, micro-trauma and degeneration. Schwartzman et al. (2017) noted that within pathological tendons there is a lack of inflammatory cells such as macrophages and neutrophils, making the correct term 'lateral tendinosis' or 'lateral epicondylalgia'.

Table 8.5 Extensor carpi radialis brevis

Muscle	Origin	Insertion	Action	Innervation
Extensor carpi radialis brevis	Humerus at the lateral epicondyle	Posterior base of the 3rd metacarpal	Extensor and abductor of the hand and wrist joint	Deep branch of the radial nerve

In a study by Olaussan et al. (2015), 177 patients were treated with 15 minutes of deep transverse friction massage at the tendon origin twice weekly for six weeks. The study included a massage group and a placebo injection group, with both groups undergoing stretching, Mills manipulation and eccentric exercise. No significant difference in outcomes was demonstrated at a one year follow up: both the control group (wait and see) and the placebo injection with physiotherapy group showed a gradual increase in success. However, Joseph et al.'s systematic review of nine studies (2012) did find some evidence of the benefit of using deep friction massage (DFM) at the elbow in combination with a Mills manipulation (as well as for supraspinatus tendinopathy) in the presence of outlet impingement and along with joint mobilisation. The authors concluded that examination of DFM as a single modality of treatment in comparison with other methods and control has not been undertaken, so its isolated efficacy has not been established. Furthermore, a Cochrane systematic review by Loew et al. (2014) demonstrated there was insufficient evidence to determine the effects of deep transverse friction on pain, improvement in grip strength and functional status for patients with lateral elbow tendinitis (or knee tendinitis). The authors also stated that the confidence intervals of the estimate of effects overlapped the null value for deep transverse friction massage in combination with physical therapy, compared with physical therapy alone, in the treatment of lateral elbow tendinitis (and knee tendinitis). Trivedi et al. (2014) concluded active release technique and myofascial release technique (described in Chapter 5) are effective in patients with chronic lateral epicondylitis, with myofascial release technique demonstrating better outcomes than active release technique in the management of chronic lateral epicondylitis. Thus, despite extensive research, there is no consensus on a universally accepted treatment method for this painful condition (Luk et al., 2014).

Special Tests

Mill's Test

The therapist palpates the athlete's lateral epicondyle with one hand while pronating the patient's forearm, fully flexing the wrist and extending the elbow. Reproduction of pain in the area of the insertion at the lateral epicondyle indicates a positive test – 100% specificity (Saroja et al., 2014).

Maudsley's Test

The therapist resists extension of the third finger of the hand, stressing the extensor digitorum muscle and tendon, while palpating the athlete's lateral epicondyle. Reproduction of pain over the lateral epicondyle of the humerus indicates a positive test.

Cozen's Test

The therapist stabilises the athlete's elbow in 90 degrees of flexion with one hand while palpating over the lateral epicondyle. The athlete's hand is moved into radial deviation and pronation. The athlete resists wrist extension in this position against the manual resistance of the therapist. A positive test is indicated if pain is reproduced in the lateral epicondyle. Cozen's test and Maudsley's test indicate 84% sensitivity and 88% sensitivity respectively and 0% specificity (Saroja et al., 2014).

Treatment Options for Tennis Elbow

After initially warming the area with effleurage techniques which should progressively get deeper and slower; start by applying direct pressure with the thumbs (or reinforced thumbs) into any trigger points (Figure 8.13). Hold for 10–30 seconds, until pain and/or a release in

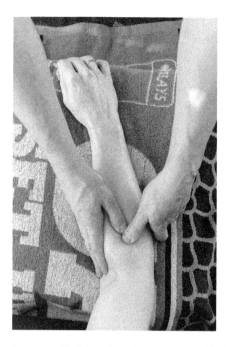

Figure 8.13 Following effleurage, use reinforced thumbs from distal to proximal in small sections to work through the extensor musculature (avoiding the insertion point).

tissue tension is felt. This can then be followed by small circular frictions to break down further adhesions. After going back to effleurage to check the area, soft tissue release can be used on the extensor muscles if deemed necessary. In more chronic cases, transverse deep friction massage can be used across the common extensor tendon near the attachment on the lateral epicondyle. Shock wave therapy, medications and ice to relieve pain can be used alongside rehabilitation exercises, accompanied with technique and training load modification which may also be necessary in some cases, prior to returning to play.

Medial Epicondylitis – Golfer's Elbow

Medial epicondylitis, also known as 'golfer's elbow' or 'thrower's elbow' (Figure 8.14), refers to the chronic tendinosis of the flexor-pronator musculature insertion on the medial epicondyle of the humerus as a result of overuse or repetitive stress (Reece & Susmarski, 2020). The flexor carpi radialis and the pronator teres (see Table 8.6) are the most commonly involved tendons in medial epicondylitis (Reece & Susmarski, 2020), although it has also been suggested all (flexor) muscles are affected equally except for palmaris longus (Kiel & Kaiser, 2020). During the acute phase there is reduced range of motion, local tenderness or pain, reduced grip strength and inflammation to the common flexor tendon near the insertion on the medial epicondyle. Repetitive activity leads to recurrent microtears within the tendon and subsequent tendinosis (Kiel & Kaiser, 2020) and has an annual incidence estimated at 1.5% (Descatha et al., 2003).

Grip strength weakness and pain during gripping is common for athletes who have suffered with medial epicondylitis. Massage may be a valuable therapy in these cases, as Molouki and colleagues (2016) discovered. In the authors' research, immediately after one session of massage to the forearm and hand, grip endurance improved ($p < 0.001$) in 44 healthy young men. Positive effects were also found in earlier research by Brooks et al. (2005). The authors revealed that 52

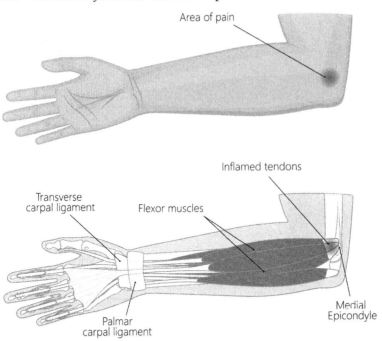

Figure 8.14 Vector illustration of Medial Epicondylitis or golfer's elbow. Used: transparency, blend mode, gradient.

Table 8.6 Flexor digitorum superficialis, pronator teres, flexor carpi radialis and flexor carpi ulnaris

Muscle	Origin	Insertion	Action	Innervation
Flexor digitorum superficialis	Medial epicondyle of humerus, coronoid process of ulna, proximal half of anterior border of radius	Sides of middle phalanges of digits 2–5	Meta- carpophalangeal and proximal interphalangeal joints of digits 2–5	Median nerve, C8–T1
Pronator teres	Humeral head, medial supracondylar ridge of humerus, coronoid process of ulna	Lateral surface of radius	Pronator of forearm and proximal radio-ulna joint	Median nerve C6–C7
Flexor carpi radialis	Medial epicondyle of humerus	Base of 2nd and 3rd metacarpals	Wrist flexion, wrist abduction	Median nerve, C6–C7
Flexor carpi ulnaris	Medial epicondyle. Ulnar head, aponeurosis from medial olecranon and upper three quarters subcutaneous border of ulna	Pisiform, hook of hamate, base of 5th metacarpals	Flexes and abducts wrist. Fixes pisiform	Ulna nerve, C8, T1

participants who received 5 minutes of massage had a greater effect ($p = 0.05$) than no massage or placebo on grip performance after fatigue, especially in the nondominant-hand group. Contrary to this, Bedford and Robbins (2016) used non-symptomatic high-level amateur and former professional racquet sports players ($n = 25$), finding the acute effects of massage (3 minutes) had no positive or negative effects on subsequent grip strength. Although these trials were on asymptomatic individuals, if massage is able to reduce painful symptoms of medial epicondylitis whilst maintaining or improving grip performance, its use should not be overlooked.

Special Test

Reverse Mill's Test

The therapist extends the athlete's elbow, wrist and fingers to stretch the common flexor tendon. The therapist supinates the forearm to increase the stretch of the tendon. A positive test is indicated if pain is reproduced over the medial epicondyle.

Treatment Options for Golfer's Elbow

Initially, effleurage to warm the area, soften adhesions, and increase local circulation, followed by petrissage to relieve tightness mobilise the tissue. Continue with deep longitudinal strokes from distal to proximal breaking down adhesion and loosening tight areas, followed by deep circular frictions to further release the superficial fascia. Trigger point therapy and soft tissue release (Figure 8.15) should be considered if necessary. Typically, other physical therapy interventions including, wrist flexor stretching, wrist flexor strengthening, ultrasound, shock wave therapy, dry needling, cross-fibre friction massage, heat and ice can all be used.

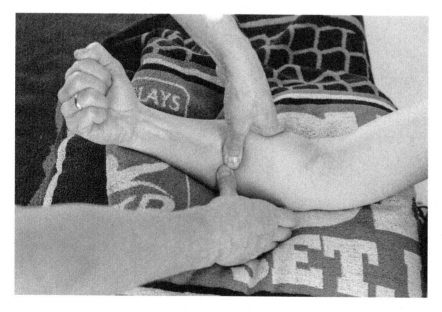

Figure 8.15 The athlete starts with a flexed wrist and makes a fist. As pressure is applied, the athlete slowly extends the wrist whilst opening the fingers. Repeat 3–5 times as necessary, with adjustments made to the position of the lock.

Shoulder Impingement

Of the 20% to 50% of people within the United Kingdom who seek shoulder pain treatment from a general practitioner, 25% of these individuals are then diagnosed with shoulder impingement syndrome (Creech & Silver, 2020). Shoulder impingement syndrome is defined as the compression of the rotator cuff (shown in Figures 8.16 and 8.17) and the subacromial bursa (Dong et al., 2015), caused by actions of shoulder including abduction, forward flexion,

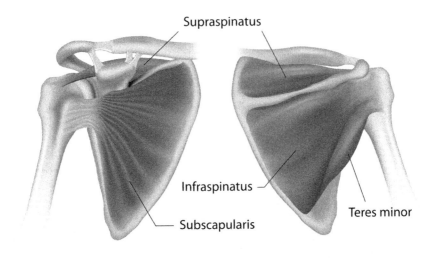

Figure 8.16 Rotator cuff anatomy.

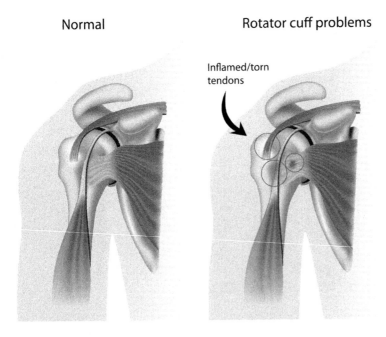

Figure 8.17 Sport injury – shoulder impingement, rotator cuff problems.

and internal rotation and normal shoulder girdle movement which result in narrowing of the subacromial space (Creech & Silver, 2020).

It is particularly prevalent in athletes who participate in sports which require repetitive overhead shoulder movements, eventually causing micro-trauma to the tendon, but affected patients are generally over age 40 and suffer from persistent pain without any known preceding trauma (Garving et al., 2017). Pain is felt across the anterior and lateral aspect of the shoulder area as the conjoint tendon of the rotator cuff gets compressed under the coracoacromial arch, causing pain to radiate down to the upper arm. The supraspinatus tendon (near its insertion at the greater tuberosity) is the most commonly implicated rotator cuff muscle in shoulder impingement. As the arm is abducted or rotated, the subacromial space width changes and the cuff becomes increasingly compressed (Khan et al., 2013). According to a study by Haveri et al. (2019), Neer's test, painful arc test and full can test form the best combination in diagnosing supraspinatus tears of any type.

Neer (1972) described the three stages of shoulder impingement as follows: Stage 1: oedema, acute inflammation and haemorrhage, age < 25, reversible; Stage 2: fibrosis and tendinitis, age 25–40, recurrent pain with activity; Stage 3: bone spurs and tendon partial or complete rupture, possible osteophyte formation, age > 40, progressive disability.

It is beyond the scope of this book to include all shoulder impingement special tests; however, some have been included.

Special Tests

Hawkins-Kennedy Test

With the elbow in 90 degrees of flexion, the examiner forward flexes the arm to 90 degrees then quickly medially rotates the shoulder (Magee, 2014). Pain over the acromion indicates subacromial impingement but may be negative in internal impingement (Cools et al., 2008). Marked rotator cuff weakness with positive impingement signs may indicate a complete cuff rupture (Koester et al., 2005).

Neer Sign

With the scapula fixed into a depressed position, this test is performed by the examiner maximally forward flexing the patient's arm (passive range of motion testing). Localised pain on the anterior shoulder suggests subacromial impingement, whereas posterior shoulder pain suggests internal impingement (Creech & Silver, 2020).

Jobe Manoeuvre (Empty Can Test)

The shoulder is abducted 90 degrees, forward flexed 30 degrees and maximally internally rotated, the elbow fully extended, and the forearm fully pronated (Jobe & Moynes, 1982).

Massage techniques have been extensively used in physical therapy practice for the treatment of shoulder pain (Karels et al., 2006). For example, Stratford et al. (1995) demonstrated that massage over a two-week period yielded improvements in abduction (mean: 42.2°, 95% CI: 24.1–60.4°), flexion (mean: 22.6°, 95% CI: 12.4–32.6°), hand behind back reach (mean: 11.0 cm further). Positive results were also found more recently, in a systematic literature review followed by a meta-analysis (Yeun, 2017) of 15 studies that included a total of 635 participants; the analysis indicated that the effect size of short-term efficacy was large and robust, supporting the hypothesis massage is an effective treatment for reducing shoulder pain.

Incorporating myofascial trigger points around the shoulder was also supported: inter-rater reliability for identification of trigger points (TP) and taut bands around the shoulder has been shown to have moderately high reliability (percentage of pairwise agreement ≥ 70%; range: 63–93%) (Bron et al., 2007), which indicates TPs should form part of the treatment plan.

Treatment Options for Shoulder Impingement

Effleurage to the pectoral area, followed by deep stroking (with reinforced fingers or the heel of the hand) should be used initially. Soft tissue release techniques can be used as long as they do not provoke shoulder pain during movement. The mid-thoracic area, latissimus dorsi and teres major (internal rotators) should be released with effleurage, petrissage, deep circular frictions and trigger point therapy. Use soft tissue release and METs on latissimus dorsi and upper trapezius. Posture, exercise selection, technique and training load/volume need to be addressed.

Plantar Heel Pain

Plantar fasciitis (PF) is soreness or tenderness of the heel that often radiates from the central part of the heel pad or the medial tubercle of the calcaneus (Figure 8.18), but may also extend

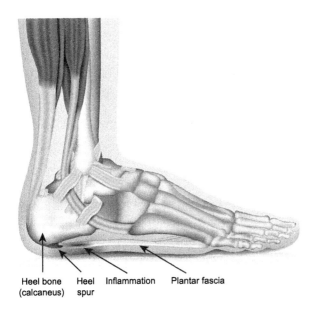

Heel bone   Heel   Inflammation   Plantar fascia
(calcaneus)   spur

Figure 8.18 Plantar fasciitis.

along the plantar fascia into the medial longitudinal arch of the foot (Landorf, 2015). It is divided into central, medial and lateral sections. It has a prevalence ranging from 4% to over 10% over the course of a lifetime (Martin et al., 2014), and accounts for 8% of all injuries in athletes in running-related sports (McPoil et al., 2008). This is unsurprising, as during each foot contact of running the plantar fascia repetitively experiences tension as high as 0.6–3.7 times the body weight, with its longitudinal strain up to 6% (Wager & Challis, 2016; McDonald et al., 2016; Chen et al., 2019).

Likely causes of plantar fasciitis are poor foot mechanics, overuse (micro-trauma) degeneration, associated muscular tightness, incorrect training principles (overload) and incorrect footwear. More recently, plantar fasciitis has been considered a degenerative pathology, similar to tendinopathy and to a chronic disease which is evident at the site of the attachment of the plantar fascia at the medial tubercle of the calcaneus (Petraglia et al., 2017). Shiotani et al. (2020) suggested that mechanical fatigue of PF is one of the causes of foot arch flattening, and in fact the change in PF stiffness at the proximal site solely explained approximately 70% of the total variance in the measures of lowering of the foot arch. This mechanical fatigue of PF and lowering of the foot arch may also increase the injury risk of proximal joints.

The best treatment modality for relieving symptoms of plantar fasciitis is still debated. Extracorporeal Shock wave therapy has demonstrated success rates of 50–65% (n = 246) (Gollwitzer et al., 2015) and a progressive exercise protocol (n = 48) performed every second day resulted in superior self-reported outcome after 3 months compared with plantar-specific stretching (Rathleff et al., 2015). In addition, Martin et al. (2014), in their summary of guidelines on heel pain/plantar fasciitis linked to the American Physical Therapy Association, stated clinicians should use manual therapy, including stretching and foot orthoses, instead of electrotherapeutic modalities to promote intermediate and long-term (1–6 months) improvements in clinical outcomes for individuals with heel pain/plantar fasciitis. Petraglia et al.'s 2017 review of the literature concluded that it had not been possible to highlight any specific diagnostic algorithm for plantar fasciitis in both recreational and elite athletes, with no evidence of different diagnostic strategies for athletes and non-athletes.

Special Test

Windlass Test

The therapist (sitting) stabilises the ankle in neutral with one hand just proximal to the first metatarsal head, then extends the first phalange while allowing the interphalangeal joint to flex. A positive test is indicated if passive extension is continued to end range or until the patient's pain is reproduced.

Standing on a stool with the metatarsal heads just off the edge of the stool, the athlete places equal weight on both feet. Again, the therapist passively extends the first phalange while allowing the interphalangeal joint to flex. A positive test is indicated if passive extension is continued to the end range or until the athlete's pain is reproduced.

Treatment Options for Plantar Fasciitis

Either in a prone or supine position, effleurage, deep stroking and petrissage to the calf area should be performed prior to addressing the plantar fascia. Once the foot has been warmed with effleurage techniques, the heel of the hand (Figure 8.19a), knuckles (Figure 8.19b), thumbs (Figure 8.19c) or a tennis ball (Figure 8.19d) can be used to loosen the fascia. It is advisable to stay away from any painful tender points under the calcaneus due to potentially aggravating any heel spur formation. Orthotics, gluteus medius strengthening and training surface modification should be considered. Training load and volume should be carefully monitored.

Muscular Cramp

Skeletal muscle cramps (MCs) are defined as sudden, involuntary and painful contractions (Minetto et al., 2013). The exact causes of muscular cramps are not fully understood, but

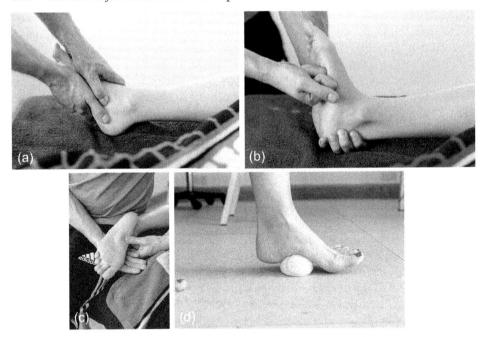

Figure 8.19 Once the foot has been warmed with effleurage techniques, release the fascia by using (a) the heel of the hand, (b) knuckles, (c) thumbs, (d) or a tennis ball.

numerous factors are thought to be involved, including muscle fatigue, prolonged muscle contractions, muscle damage, restricted muscle blood flow, diabetes, dehydration and hyperthermia (Katzberg, 2015). Traditionally it has been assumed that depletion of the extracellular volume (dehydration) is the main cause of cramp; however, it has been reported that 69% of MCs occur in subjects that are well hydrated and sufficiently supplemented with electrolytes (Jung et al., 2005).

The theory of altered neuromuscular control suggests that hyperexcitability of the motoneuron pool causes sustained motoneuron firing (Schwellnus, 2009). This hyperexcitability results from an imbalance between increased muscle-spindle activity and reduced golgi tendon organ feedback and is believed to stem from neuromuscular overload and fatigue (Miller et al., 2010; Nelson & Churilla, 2016; Panza et al., 2017; Jahic & Begic, 2018) rather than dehydration or electrolyte deficits. In agreement, Giuriato et al.'s (2018) review of 69 manuscripts suggested that action potentials during a muscle cramp are generated in the motoneuron soma, likely accompanied by an imbalance between the rising excitatory drive from the muscle spindles 1a and the decreasing inhibitory drive from the golgi tendon organs.

Treatment Options for Muscular Cramp

Lifestyle modification, treatment of underlying conditions, stretching, B-complex vitamins, diltiazem, mexiletine, carbamazepine, tetrahydrocannabinoid, levetiracetam and quinine sulphate have all shown some evidence for treatment (Katzberg, 2015). In addition, Jahic and Begic (2018) recommended treatment and prevention strategies for MC including electrical cramp induction, Kinesio taping and compression garments, massage therapy, electrolyte supplementation and hydration, corrective exercise, stretching, quinine, pickle juice and hyperventilation strategies. It is worth noting that if any athlete has repeated intermittent muscle spasms following brief episodes of exertion, they should be referred to their physician, as underlying medical conditions such as paroxysmal dyskinesias may be present (attacks are triggered by an abrupt movement or an increase of speed, amplitude or strength, the sudden addition of new actions during ongoing steady movements or a change in direction) (Manso-Calderón, 2019).

Exertional Rhabdomyolysis

Exertional rhabdomyolysis is a clinical syndrome which occurs following excessive strenuous unaccustomed exercise, including endurance and ultra-endurance events (Rojas-Valverde et al., 2020), gym-based 'spin' classes (Brogan et al., 2017), 'Cross-Fit' exercise (Meyer et al., 2018; Hopkins et al., 2019) and tennis (Henderson et al., 2019). Extensive damage to the muscle fibres can occur (delayed onset muscle soreness) and if this pain is severe, large amounts of intracellular muscle content are released into the blood stream. This content can include, for instance, creatine kinase (CK), lactate dehydrogenase (LDH) and myoglobin, which all have to be cleared by the kidneys, leading to oxidative stress and potentially acute renal failure (Chavez et al., 2016; Cabral et al., 2020). Other causes of rhabdomyolysis are numerous, and can include direct muscle injury, unaccustomed exercise, ischemia (crush injuries), extreme temperatures, electrolyte abnormalities, endocrinological conditions, genetic disorders, auto-immune disorders, infections, drugs, toxins and venoms (Rawson et al., 2017).

References

Ahmad, Z., Siddiqui, N., Malik, S.S., Abdus-Samee, M., Tytherleigh-Strong, G. and Rushton, N., 2013. Lateral epicondylitis: A review of pathology and management. *The Bone & Joint Journal, 95*(9), pp. 1158–1164.

Antonio, S., Wolfgang, G., Robert, H., Fullerton, B. and Carla, S., 2013. The anatomical and functional relation between gluteus maximus and fascia lata. *Journal of Bodywork and Movement Therapies, 17*(4), pp. 512–517.

Årøen, A., Helgø, D., Granlund, O.G. and Bahr, R., 2004. Contralateral tendon rupture risk is increased in individuals with a previous Achilles tendon rupture. *Scandinavian Journal of Medicine & Science in Sports, 14*(1), pp. 30–33.

Ayan, A. and Örsçelik, A., 2020. Bilateral Tibial stress injuries in recreational athletes of Army. *Spor Hekimliği Dergisi, 55*(1), pp. 014–020.

Aysin, I.K., Askin, A., Mete, B.D., Guvendi, E., Aysin, M. and Kocyigit, H., 2018. Investigation of the relationship between anterior knee pain and chondromalacia patellae and patellofemoral malalignment. *The Eurasian Journal of Medicine, 50*(1), p. 28.

Barton, C., Pattison, F. and Morrisey, D., 2014. Combining massage with stretching increases the short-term flexibility of the fascia lata complex: A repeated measures study. *Journal of Science and Medicine in Sport, 18*, p. e74.

Bayliss, A.J., Weatherholt, A.M., Crandall, T.T., Farmer, D.L., McConnell, J.C., Crossley, K.M. and Warden, S.J., 2016. Achilles tendon material properties are greater in the jump leg of jumping athletes. *Journal of Musculoskeletal & Neuronal Interactions, 16*(2), p. 105.

Beals, C. and Flanigan, D., 2013. A review of treatments for iliotibial band syndrome in the athletic population. *Journal of Sports Medicine, 2013*, p. 367169. https://doi.org/10.1155/2013/367169

Bedford, S. and Robbins, D., 2016. The acute effects of massage are not detrimental to grip strength in sub-elite racquet players. *Medicine & Science in Tennis, 21*(1), pp. 24–27.

Bojsen-Møller, J., Magnusson, S.P., Rasmussen, L.R., Kjaer, M. and Aagaard, P., 2005. Muscle performance during maximal isometric and dynamic contractions is influenced by the stiffness of the tendinous structures. *Journal of Applied Physiology, 99*(3), pp. 986–994.

Brogan, M., Ledesma, R., Coffino, A. and Chander, P., 2017. Freebie rhabdomyolysis: a public health concern. Spin class-induced rhabdomyolysis. *The American Journal of Medicine*, *130*(4), pp. 484–487.

Bron, C., Franssen, J., Wensing, M. and Oostendorp, R.A., 2007. Interrater reliability of palpation of myofascial trigger points in three shoulder muscles. *Journal of Manual & Manipulative Therapy*, *15*(4), pp. 203–215.

Brooks, C.P., Woodruff, L.D., Wright, L.L. and Donatelli, R., 2005. The immediate effects of manual massage on power-grip performance after maximal exercise in healthy adults. *Journal of Alternative & Complementary Medicine: Research on Paradigm, Practice, and Policy*, *11*(6), pp. 1093–1101.

Cabral, B.M.I., Edding, S.N., Portocarrero, J.P. and Lerma, E.V., 2020. Rhabdomyolysis. *Disease-a-Month*, p. 101015.

Chaves, P., Simoes, D., Paco, M., Pinho, F., Duarte, J.A. and Ribeiro, F., 2017. Cyriax's deep friction massage application parameters: Evidence from a cross-sectional study with physiotherapists. *Musculoskeletal Science and Practice*, *32*, pp. 92–97.

Chavez, L.O., Leon, M., Einav, S. and Varon, J., 2016. Beyond muscle destruction: a systematic review of rhabdomyolysis for clinical practice. *Critical Care*, *20*(1), p. 135.

Chen, T.L.W., Wong, D.W.C., Wang, Y., Lin, J. and Zhang, M., 2019. Foot arch deformation and plantar fascia loading during running with rearfoot strike and forefoot strike: A dynamic finite element analysis. *Journal of Biomechanics*, *83*, pp. 260–272.

Cools, A.M., Cambier, D. and Witvrouw, E.E., 2008. Screening the athlete's shoulder for impingement symptoms: A clinical reasoning algorithm for early detection of shoulder pathology. *British Journal of Sports Medicine*, *42*(8), pp. 628–635.

Creech, J.A. and Silver, S., 2020. Shoulder impingement syndrome. In: Creech, J.A. and Silver, S. (eds.), *StatPearls [Internet]*. Treasure Island, FL: StatPearls Publishing. Available from: https://www.ncbi.nlm.nih.gov/books/NBK554518/

Descatha, A., Leclerc, A., Chastang, J.F. and Roquelaure, Y., 2003. Medial epicondylitis in occupational settings: Prevalence, incidence and associated risk factors. *Journal of Occupational and Environmental Medicine*, *45*(9), p. 993.

Dong, W., Goost, H., Lin, X.B., Burger, C., Paul, C., Wang, Z.L., Zhang, T.Y., Jiang, Z.C., Welle, K. and Kabir, K., 2015. Treatments for shoulder impingement syndrome: A PRISMA systematic review and network meta-analysis. *Medicine*, *94*(10), p. e510. https://doi.org/10.1097/MD.0000000000000510

Fredericson, M. and Yoon, K., 2006. Physical examination and patellofemoral pain syndrome. *American Journal of Physical Medicine & Rehabilitation*, *85*(3), pp. 234–243.

Friede, M.C., Klauser, A., Fink, C. and Csapo, R., 2020. Stiffness of the iliotibial band and associated muscles in runner's knee: Assessing the effects of physiotherapy through ultrasound shear wave elastography. *Physical Therapy in Sport*, *45*, pp. 126–134.

Garving, C., Jakob, S., Bauer, I., Nadjar, R. and Brunner, U.H., 2017. Impingement syndrome of the shoulder. *Deutsches Ärzteblatt International*, *114*(45), p. 765.

Giuriato, G., Pedrinolla, A., Schena, F. and Venturelli, M., 2018. Muscle cramps: A comparison of the two-leading hypothesis. *Journal of Electromyography and Kinesiology*, *41*, pp.89–95.

Gollwitzer, H., Saxena, A., DiDomenico, L.A., Galli, L., Bouché, R.T., Caminear, D.S., Fullem, B., Vester, J.C., Horn, C., Banke, I.J. and Burgkart, R., 2015. Clinically relevant effectiveness of focused extracorporeal shock wave therapy in the treatment of chronic plantar fasciitis: A randomized, controlled multicenter study. *JBJS*, *97*(9), pp.701–708.

Hamstra-Wright, K.L., Bliven, K.C. and Bay, C., 2015. Risk factors for medial tibial stress syndrome in physically active individuals such as runners and military personnel: A systematic review and meta-analysis. *British Journal of Sports Medicine*. Mar 1, *49*(6), 362–369.

Haveri, S., Uppin, R.B. and Patil, K., 2019. The diagnostic value of the combination of clinical tests for the diagnosis of supraspinatus tendon tears. *Indian Journal of Health Sciences and Biomedical Research (KLEU)*, *12*(1), p. 91.

Henderson, K.D., Manspeaker, S.A. and Stubblefield, Z., 2019. Exertional Rhabdomyolysis in a women's tennis athlete: A case report. *International Journal of Athletic Therapy and Training*, *24*(4), pp. 156–159.

Hodgson, R.J., O'Connor, P.J. and Grainger, A.J., 2012. Tendon and ligament imaging. *The British Journal of Radiology*, *85*(1016), pp. 1157–1172.

Hopkins, B.S., Li, D., Svet, M., Kesavabhotla, K. and Dahdaleh, N.S., 2019. CrossFit and rhabdomyolysis: A case series of 11 patients presenting at a single academic institution. *Journal of Science and Medicine in Sport*, *22*(7), pp. 758–762.

Jahic, D. and Begic, E., 2018. Exercise-associated muscle cramp-doubts about the cause. *Materia Socio-Medica*, *30*(1), p. 67.

Jobe, F.W. and Moynes, D.R., 1982. Delineation of diagnostic criteria and a rehabilitation program for rotator cuff injuries. *The American Journal of Sports Medicine*, *10*(6), pp. 336–339.

Joseph, M.F., Taft, K., Moskwa, M. and Denegar, C.R., 2012. Deep friction massage to treat tendinopathy: A systematic review of a classic treatment in the face of a new paradigm of understanding. *Journal of Sport Rehabilitation*, *21*(4), pp. 343–353.

Jung, A.P., Bishop, P.A., Al-Nawwas, A. and Dale, R.B., 2005. Influence of hydration and electrolyte supplementation on incidence and time to onset of exercise-associated muscle cramps. *Journal of Athletic Training*, *40*(2), p. 71.

Karels, C.H., Polling, W., Bierma-Zeinstra, S.M., Burdorf, A., Verhagen, A.P. and Koes, B.W., 2006. Treatment of arm, neck, and/or shoulder complaints in physical therapy practice. *Spine*, *31*(17), pp. E584–E589.

Katzberg, H.D., 2015. Neurogenic muscle cramps. *Journal of Neurology*, *262*(8), pp. 1814–1821.

Khan, Y., Nagy, M.T., Malal, J. and Waseem, M., 2013. Suppl 3: The Painful Shoulder: Shoulder Impingement Syndrome. *The Open Orthopaedics Journal*, *7*, p. 347.

Kiel, J. and Kaiser, K., 2020. Golfer's Elbow. In: *StatPearls [Internet]*. Treasure Island, FL: StatPearls Publishing. Available from: https://www.ncbi.nlm.nih.gov/books/NBK519000/

Koester, M.C., George, M.S. and Kuhn, J.E., 2005. Shoulder impingement syndrome. *The American Journal of Medicine*, *118*(5), pp. 452–455.

Landorf, K.B., 2015. Plantar heel pain and plantar fasciitis. *BMJ Clinical Evidence*, *2015*, p. 1111.

Loew, L.M., Brosseau, L., Tugwell, P., Wells, G.A., Welch, V., Shea, B., Poitras, S., De Angelis, G. and Rahman, P., 2014. Deep transverse friction massage for treating lateral elbow or lateral knee tendinitis. *Cochrane Database of Systematic Reviews*, (11), CD003528. https://doi.org/10.1002/14651858.CD003528.pub2

Longo, U.G., Ronga, M. and Maffulli, N., 2018. Achilles tendinopathy. *Sports Medicine and Arthroscopy Review*, *26*(1), pp. 16–30.

Lopes, A.D., Hespanhol, L.C., Yeung, S.S. and Costa, L.O.P., 2012. What are the main running-related musculoskeletal injuries? *Sports Medicine*, *42*(10), pp. 891–905.

Lorimer, A.V. and Hume, P.A., 2016. Stiffness as a risk factor for Achilles tendon injury in running athletes. *Sports Medicine*, *46*(12), pp. 1921–1938.

Louw, M. and Deary, C., 2014. The biomechanical variables involved in the aetiology of iliotibial band syndrome in distance runners – A systematic review of the literature. *Physical Therapy in Sport*, *15*(1), pp. 64–75.

Luk, J.K., Tsang, R.C. and Leung, H.B., 2014. Lateral epicondylalgia: Midlife crisis of a tendon. *Hong Kong Medical Journal*, *20*(2), pp. 145–51.

Maffulli, N., Sharma, P. and Luscombe, K.L., 2004. Achilles tendinopathy: Aetiology and management. *Journal of the Royal Society of Medicine*, *97*(10), pp. 472–476.

Magee, D.J., 2014. *Orthopaedic physical assessment-E-Book*. Missouri: Elsevier Health Sciences.

Manso-Calderón, R., 2019. The spectrum of paroxysmal dyskinesias. *Future Neurology*, *14*(3), p. FNL26.

Martin, R.L., Davenport, T.E., Reischl, S.F., McPoil, T.G., Matheson, J.W., Wukich, D.K., McDonough, C.M., Altman, R.D., Beattie, P., Cornwall, M. and Davis, I., 2014. Heel pain

– plantar fasciitis: Revision 2014. *Journal of Orthopaedic & Sports Physical Therapy*, *44*(11), pp. A1–A33.

McDonald, K.A., Stearne, S.M., Alderson, J.A., North, I., Pires, N.J. and Rubenson, J., 2016. The role of arch compression and metatarsophalangeal joint dynamics in modulating plantar fascia strain in running. *PloS One*, *11*(4), p. e0152602.

McNamara, W., Sunwoo, J., Ho, G., Lindsay, B., Miller, R. and Cole, B., 2019. Treatment of reduced ankle range of motion in medial tibial stress syndrome using an investigational lower leg device. *Journal of Science and Medicine in Sport*, *22*, p. S95.

McPoil, T.G., Martin, R.L., Cornwall, M.W., Wukich, D.K., Irrgang, J.J. and Godges, J.J., 2008. Heel pain – plantar fasciitis. *Journal of Orthopaedic & Sports Physical Therapy*, *38*(4), pp. A1–A18.

Meyer, M., Sundaram, S. and Schafhalter-Zoppoth, I., 2018. Exertional and cross-fit induced rhabdomyolysis. *Clinical Journal of Sport Medicine: Official Journal of the Canadian Academy of Sport Medicine*, *28*(6), pp. e92–e94.

Miller, K.C., Mack, G.W., Knight, K.L., Hopkins, J.T., Draper, D.O., Fields, P.J. and Hunter, I., 2010. Reflex inhibition of electrically induced muscle cramps in hypo-hydrated humans. *Medicine & Science in Sports & Exercise*, *42*(5), pp. 953–961.

Minetto, M.A., Holobar, A., Botter, A. and Farina, D., 2013. Origin and development of muscle cramps. *Exercise and Sport Sciences Reviews*, *41*(1), pp. 3–10.

Moen, M.H., Tol, J.L., Weir, A., Steunebrink, M. and De Winter, T.C., 2009. Medial tibial stress syndrome. *Sports Medicine*, *39*(7), pp. 523–546.

Molouki, A., Hosseini, S.M., Rustaee, M. and Tabatabaee, S.M., 2016. The immediate effects of manual massage of forearm on power-grip strength and endurance in healthy young men. *Journal of Chiropractic Medicine*, *15*(2), pp. 112–120.

Nath, J., 2015. Effect of hip abductor strengthening among non-professional cyclists with iliotibial band friction syndrome. *International Journal of Physiotherapy and Research*, *3*(1), pp. 894–904.

Neer, C.S. II., 1972. Anterior acromioplasty for the chronic impingement syndrome in the shoulder: a preliminary report. *Journal of Bone and Joint Surgery*, *54*, pp. 41–50.

Nelson, N.L. and Churilla, J.R., 2016. A narrative review of exercise-associated muscle cramps: Factors that contribute to neuromuscular fatigue and management implications. *Muscle & nerve*, *54*(2), pp. 177–185.

Noehren, B., Schmitz, A., Hempel, R., Westlake, C. and Black, W., 2014. Assessment of strength, flexibility, and running mechanics in men with iliotibial band syndrome. *Journal of Orthopaedic & Sports Physical Therapy*, *44*(3), pp. 217–222.

Olaussen, M., Holmedal, Ø., Mdala, I., Brage, S. and Lindbæk, M., 2015. Corticosteroid or placebo injection combined with deep transverse friction massage, mills manipulation, stretching and eccentric exercise for acute lateral epicondylitis: a randomised, controlled trial. *BMC Musculoskeletal Disorders*, *16*(1), p. 122.

Panken, A.M., Heymans, M.W., Van Oort, L. and Verhagen, A.P., 2015. Clinical prognostic factors for patients with anterior knee pain in physical therapy; a systematic review. *International Journal of Sports Physical Therapy*, *10*(7), p. 929.

Panza, G., Stadler, J., Murray, D., Lerma, N., Barrett, T., Pettit-Mee, R. and Edwards, J.E., 2017. Acute passive static stretching and cramp threshold frequency. *Journal of Athletic Training*, *52*(10), pp. 918–924.

Petraglia, F., Ramazzina, I. and Costantino, C., 2017. Plantar fasciitis in athletes: diagnostic and treatment strategies. A systematic review. *Muscles, Ligaments and Tendons Journal*, *7*(1), p. 107.

Rathleff, M.S., Mølgaard, C.M., Fredberg, U., Kaalund, S., Andersen, K.B., Jensen, T.T., Aaskov, S. and Olesen, J.L., 2015. High-load strength training improves outcome in patients with plantar fasciitis: A randomized controlled trial with 12-month follow-up. *Scandinavian Journal of Medicine & Science in Sports*, *25*(3), pp. e292–e300.

Rawson, E.S., Clarkson, P.M. and Tarnopolsky, M.A., 2017. Perspectives on exertional rhabdomyolysis. *Sports Medicine*, *47*(1), pp. 33–49.

Reece, C.L. and Susmarski, A., 2020. Medial Epicondylitis. In *StatPearls [Internet]*. Treasure Island, FL: StatPearls Publishing.

Rojas-Valverde, D., Sánchez-Ureña, B., Crowe, J., Timón, R. and Olcina, G.J., 2020. Exertional rhabdomyolysis and acute kidney injury in endurance sports: A systematic review. *European Journal of Sport Science*, pp. 1–14.

Rothermich, M.A., Glaviano, N.R., Li, J. and Hart, J.M., 2015. Patellofemoral pain: epidemiology, pathophysiology, and treatment options. *Clinics in Sports Medicine*, 34(2), pp. 313–327.

Sanchis-Alfonso, V., Ramírez-Fuentes, C., Roselló-Sastre, E., Dye, S.F. and Teitge, R.A., 2020. Pathophysiology of anterior knee pain. In: Dejour, D., Zaffagnini, S., Arendt, E., Sillanpää, P. and Dirisamer F. (eds), *Patellofemoral pain, instability, and arthritis* (pp. 93–116). Berlin, Heidelberg: Springer. https://doi.org/10.1007/978-3-662-61097-8_8

Saroja, G., Aseer, P.A.L. and Venkata Sai, P.M., 2014. Diagnostic accuracy of provocative tests in lateral epicondylitis. *International Journal of Physiotherapy and Research*, 2(6), pp. 815–823.

Schwarzman, G., Watson, J.N. and Hutchinson, M.R., 2017. Lateral epicondylopathy (Aka. tennis elbow): A review of current concepts and treatment. *Annals of Sports Medicine and Research*, 4(5), p. 1117.

Schwellnus, M.P., 2009. Cause of exercise associated muscle cramps (EAMC)—altered neuromuscular control, dehydration or electrolyte depletion? *British Journal of Sports Medicine*, 43(6), pp. 401–408.

Shiotani, H., Mizokuchi, T., Yamashita, R., Naito, M. and Kawakami, Y., 2020. Acute effects of long-distance running on mechanical and morphological properties of the human plantar fascia. *Scandinavian Journal of Medicine & Science in Sports*, 30(8), pp. 1360–1368.

Stratford, P., Gill, C., Westaway, M. and Binkley, J., 1995. Assessing disability and change on individual patients: A report of a patient specific measure. *Physiotherapy Canada*, 47(4), pp. 258–263.

Taunton, J.E., Ryan, M.B., Clement, D.B., McKenzie, D.C., Lloyd-Smith, D.R. and Zumbo, B.D., 2002. A retrospective case-control analysis of 2002 running injuries. *British Journal of Sports Medicine*, 36(2), pp. 95–101.

Trivedi, P., Sathiyavani, D., Nambi, G., Khuman, R., Shah, K. and Bhatt, P., 2014. Comparison of active release technique and myofascial release technique on pain, grip strength & functional performance in patients with chronic lateral epicondylitis. *International Journal of Physiotherapy and Research*, 2(3), pp. 488–494.

Trofa, D.P., Miller, J.C., Jang, E.S., Woode, D.R., Greisberg, J.K. and Vosseller, J.T., 2017. Professional athletes' return to play and performance after operative repair of an Achilles tendon rupture. *The American Journal of Sports Medicine*, 45(12), pp. 2864–2871.

Van der Worp, M.P., van der Horst, N., de Wijer, A., Backx, F.J. and Nijhuis-van der Sanden, M.W., 2012. Iliotibial band syndrome in runners. *Sports Medicine*, 42(11), pp. 969–992.

Ververidis, A.N., Touzopoulos, P., Drosos, G.I., Tilkeridis, K.E. and Kazakos, K.I., 2016. Percutaneous repair of the Achilles tendon rupture in athletic population. *Journal of Orthopaedics*, 13(1), pp. 57–61.

Wager, J.C. and Challis, J.H., 2016. Elastic energy within the human plantar aponeurosis contributes to arch shortening during the push-off phase of running. *Journal of Biomechanics*, 49(5), pp. 704–709.

Wang, T.G., Jan, M.H., Lin, K.H. and Wang, H.K., 2006. Assessment of stretching of the iliotibial tract with Ober and modified Ober tests: An ultrasonographic study. *Archives of Physical Medicine and Rehabilitation*, 87(10), pp. 1407–1411.

Weinreb, J.H., Sheth, C., Apostolakos, J., McCarthy, M.B., Barden, B., Cote, M.P. and Mazzocca, A.D., 2014. Tendon structure, disease, and imaging. *Muscles, Ligaments and Tendons Journal*, 4(1), p. 66.

Willett, G.M., Keim, S.A., Shostrom, V.K. and Lomneth, C.S., 2016. An anatomic investigation of the Ober test. *The American Journal of Sports Medicine*, 44(3), pp. 696–701. doi:10.1177/0363546515621762

Yeun, Y.R., 2017. Effectiveness of massage therapy for shoulder pain: A systematic review and meta-analysis. *Journal of Physical Therapy Science*, 29(5), pp. 936–940.

9 Back Pain and Spinal Curvatures

Low Back Pain

There are a number of potential causes of low back pain (LBP), of which one plausible explanation is mechanical damage. Mechanical damage will occur if the posterior loading associated with the lumbar lordosis exceeds the load tolerance of the tissues (Sorensen et al., 2015). The muscles of the lower back are shown in Figure 9.1.

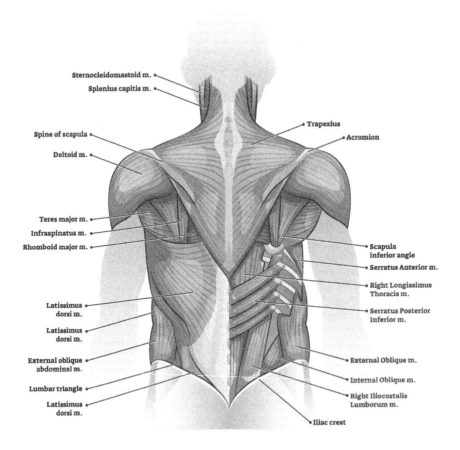

Figure 9.1 Muscles of the back.

DOI: 10.4324/9781003104803-9

A number of studies using massage as a treatment modality for low back pain have demonstrated positive results, including Kumar et al.'s (2013) analysis of systematic reviews on the effectiveness of massage therapy for the treatment of non-specific low back pain. The authors concluded that the primary research informing these systematic reviews was generally of weak quality, but the findings did indicate massage may be an effective treatment option when compared to placebo and some active treatment options (such as relaxation), especially in the short term. In addition, Daneau et al. (2019) demonstrated that pain perception (p = 0.004) was reduced after a single 30-minute massage on 36 participants with chronic lower back pain, but massage yielded no significant effect on fatigue-related physiological variables. In agreement, an Ottawa panel of evidence-based clinical practice guidelines on therapeutic massage for low back pain (Brosseau et al., 2012) concluded massage interventions are effective, when combined with therapeutic exercise and education, in providing short term improvement of sub-acute and chronic lower back pain symptoms, decreasing disability immediately post-treatment and providing short-term relief. Further positive results indicated that adults (m age = 39.6 years) with low back pain of at least 6 months in duration who received two 30-minute massage or relaxation therapy sessions per week for 5 weeks reportedly experienced less pain, depression and anxiety, and their sleep improved. They also showed improved trunk and pain flexion performance, and their serotonin and dopamine levels were higher (Hernandez-Reif et al., 2001). Contrary to these positive findings, Furlan et al.'s (2015) systematic review on massage for low back pain concluded the authors had very little confidence that massage is an effective treatment for LBP. Acute, sub-acute and chronic LBP had improvements in pain outcomes with massage only in the short-term follow-up. Functional improvement was observed in participants with sub-acute and chronic LBP when compared with inactive controls, but only in the short-term follow-up. There were only minor adverse effects with massage.

Elder et al. (2017) enrolled 104 chronic low back pain patients, of which 85 and 76 completed 12 and 24 weeks of data collection, respectively. Group means improved at 12 weeks for all outcomes and at 24 weeks for Short Form Health Survey version 2.0's (SF-36v2)'s physical component summary and bodily pain domain. Of those with clinically improved disability at 12 weeks, 75% were still clinically improved at 24 weeks ($p < 0.01$). For SF-36v2 physical and mental component summaries, 55.4% and 43.4%, respectively, showed clinically meaningful improvement at 12 weeks, and 46.1% and 30.3% at 24 weeks. For the bodily pain domain, 49.4% were clinically improved at 12 weeks, and 40% at 24 weeks. Therefore, this study provides some encouraging results, indicating that massage may have some long-lasting effects on chronic low back pain. In addition, results from a study using 16 elite female wrestlers demonstrated that a combination therapy of massage and lumbopelvic stability training had significantly greater effects in reducing pain perception (45–51%), improving pain pressure threshold (15–25%) and increasing tissue blood flow (131–152%) than massage therapy alone ($p < 0.001$) (Joseph et al., 2018).

Frequently, in conjunction with massage, athletes use a number of other modalities including rehabilitation exercises, manipulation, traction, mobilisations, electrical stimulation devices, acupuncture (dry needling) and medication to relieve low back pain. However, as Thompson et al. (2020) implied, there is apparent uncertainty over which pool of interventions constitute the most effective options for treating non-specific chronic low back pain (CLBP), indicating there is a need for a stronger evidence base.

Treatment Options for Non-Specific Low Back Pain

Begin with effleurage to the lower back and gluteal region, followed by petrissage to thoroughly warm and mobilise the area. This can be followed by deeper stroking techniques across the lower back in various directions. Trigger points (using ischemic compression) can be addressed, particularly in the quadratus lumborum area (Figure 9.2a) and gluteus medius (Figure 9.2b). Mobility exercises and stretching may also assist in rehabilitation. Athletes who experience neurological symptoms or any other unexplained pathologies need to be referred to the appropriate medical practitioner.

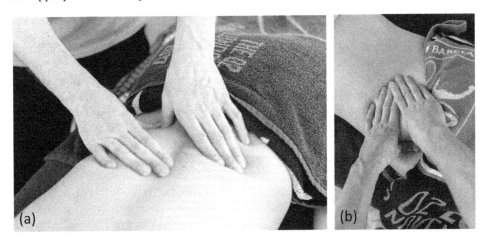

Figure 9.2 Trigger points (using ischemic compression) can be addressed, particularly in the quadratus lumborum area (a) and gluteus medius (b).

Spinal Curvatures

The transition to a vertically oriented spine from a semi-orthograde spinal orientation during human evolution resulted in the gravity vector considerably realigning from its original axis, a change that has led to dramatic kinetic and kinematic changes in the human spine (Hay et al., 2015). This, over time, has led to the spinal curvatures we recognise today (Figure 9.3).

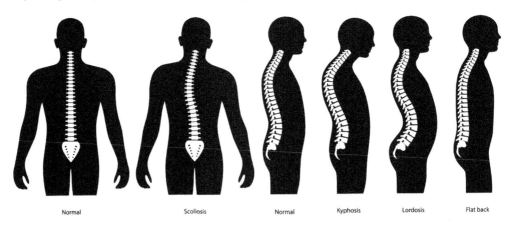

Figure 9.3 Spinal deformity types. White spine on a black body. Anterior view and lateral view. Vector illustration.

The main curvatures are lumbar lordosis (LL), thoracic kyphosis and scoliosis, all of which are described below.

Lumbar Lordosis

The definition of lumbar lordosis is widely debated in the literature, as different reference points have been used as measurements. Frenkel et al. (2018) proposed that a standardised definition of LL, from the superior endplate of L-1 to the superior endplate of S-1, should be adopted. For simplicity, lumbar lordosis is defined as an excessive inward curve of the spine. The spine's natural curves position the head over the pelvis, working as shock absorbers to distribute mechanical stress during ambulation and maintain our centre of mass.

Three studies involving 1,657 participants with lumbar lordosis provided data for a meta-analysis (Sadler et al., 2017). This study revealed a significant association between a reduction in lumbar lordosis and the risk of developing lower back pain (OR = 0.73, 95% CI 0.55–0.98, $p = 0.034$) or a 37% greater likelihood of developing lower back pain in people with restricted lumbar lordosis. However, Chun et al.'s (2017) meta-analysis demonstrated a strong relationship between low back pain and decreased lumbar lordotic curvature. Additionally, in a further study linking lumbar lordosis with lower back pain, Sorensen et al.'s (2015) results indicated that standing in a more lumbar lordotic posture may be a risk factor for low back pain development during prolonged periods of standing. There were 24 (42%) pain developers and 33 (58%) non-pain developers. Lumbar lordosis was significantly larger in pain developers compared to non-pain developers (mean difference = 4.4°; 95%. The correlation coefficient between lumbar lordosis and maximum pain was 0.46 ($p = 0.02$). The authors commented that it is reasonable to propose that in back-healthy people the degree of lumbar lordosis may contribute to an increase in susceptibility for LBP symptoms during prolonged standing.

A common feature of lumbar hyper-lordosis (excessive curvature of the lumbar spine) is increased stiffness of the anterior supporting structures of the thigh, hip and lumbar spine, resulting in a compensatory exaggerated anterior pelvic tilt with lumbar extension motion during knee flexion or prone hip extension (Sahrmann, 2002). Other causes include an imbalance between trunk muscles (Kim et al., 2006) and excessive foot pronation, leading to an internally rotated tibial and femoral position which may encourage an anterior pelvic tilt (Barwick et al., 2012). Although less common, a flattened lumbar lordosis can occur and has been associated with pelvic retroversion due to increased activation of trained abdominal and gluteal muscles (Grabara, 2015). Areas that should be massaged and stretched on athletes with a hyper-lordotic curvature should include the quadriceps, hip flexors, gluteals and erector spinae muscle group. The gluteals, hamstrings and abdominals should be strengthened.

Kyphosis

Kyphosis is curvature of the spine that causes the top of the back to appear more rounded than normal, with a curve of more than 45 degrees considered excessive. With increased kyphosis at the thoracic spine, anterior longitudinal ligament and upper abdominal muscles are shortened and the anterior aspect of vertebral bodies is compressed, leading to increases in intradiscal pressures (Singla & Veqar, 2017).

Although there are some medical conditions which may cause a thoracic curvature (e.g. Scheuermann's kyphosis, osteoporosis, ankylosing spondylosis), in the general and athletic population, rounded shoulders and forward head posture could be a result of long-term operation of computers which induce unbalanced kinematics of muscles around the neck, chest and back (Lv et al., 2016). Some sports, such as cycling, tennis and hockey, require the athlete to be in a forward flexed position for long durations. This was demonstrated by Rajabi et al. (2012), who concluded thoracic kyphosis was significantly increased in adolescent female field hockey players ($n = 37$) and was found to be associated with the cumulative number of years of hockey participation.

High training loads and frequently repeated unilateral movement patterns during sports training can have an impact on the curvatures of the spine. In kyphotic athletes, therapists should concentrate massage and stretching around the pectorals and latissimus dorsi (internal rotators). The use of a foam roller to encourage thoracic extension, strengthening the midback muscles (mid and lower trapezius, rhomboids) and addressing poor habitual posture and repetitive movement patterns through corrective movements and training loads, accompanied by restoration of good biomechanical alignment, should be a priority.

Scoliosis

Thoracic scoliosis can cause the chest to twist into an unusual position, which causes the chest, pelvis and hips to become misaligned (Purnama et al., 2018). Jandric (2015) defined scoliosis as

> a lateral curvature of the spinal column in the coronal plane. However, the disorder actually occurs in three dimensions (3D): apart from a lateral curvature in the coronal plane, there is also rotation (motion around the longitudinal axis in the transverse plane) and torsion (twisting of a part of a vertebral body towards another one, and a change of profile in the sagittal plane).

In the athletic population, length of training time (especially at an early age), high volume, one-sided and asymmetrical sports, such as rowing, fencing, tennis, track and field and throwing disciplines, may cause hypertonicity of the muscles on the dominant side of the body, leading to habitual scoliosis. Therefore, massage should be concentrated on these areas to restore muscle length and release tension where possible. Additionally, exercises on the sides of the arms and legs that are not dominant are required to maintain muscle balance.

Neural Tension and Piriformis Syndrome

The piriformis muscle, as shown in Figure 9.4, has a broad origin at the anterior sacral vertebrae and runs laterally through the greater sciatic foramen. It then inserts on the piriformis fossa at the greater trochanter of the proximal femur (Jankovic et al., 2013). Functionally it is an external rotator of the hip during extension, abductor of the hip at 60 degrees, and internal rotation during 90 degrees of flexion at hip joint (Table 9.1).

Piriformis syndrome is a clinical condition of sciatic nerve entrapment at the level of the ischial tuberosity (Hicks & Varacallo, 2017). Its presenting symptom invariably is gluteal pain which occurs in 98% of cases. The secondary sciatic nerve entrapment is symptomatic in 82% of cases and here patients complain of pain and paraesthesia in the buttock, hip and posterior thigh. Leg pain is less commonly seen and is the presenting symptom in 60% of cases (Younus & Kelly, 2020). The piriformis can be stressed due to poor body mechanics in a chronic condition or an acute injury with the forceful internal rotation of the hip (Hicks & Varacallo, 2017). One case study report (Tchorowska & Wilk, 2020) revealed twiceweekly 45-minute massages over eight treatments to the lower back, gluteal and selected

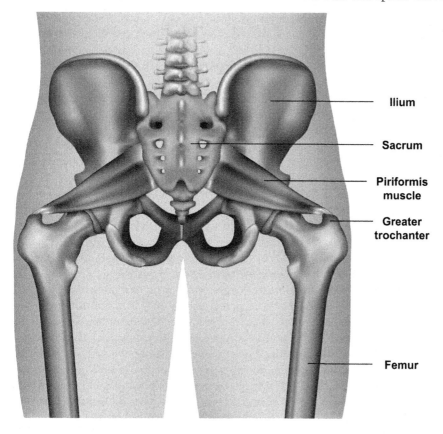

Figure 9.4 Piriformis muscle (3D medical vector illustration).

Table 9.1 Piriformis

Muscle	Origin	Insertion	Action	Innervation
Piriformis	Anterior aspect of the sacrum. Sacrotuberous ligament. Periphery of the greater sciatic notch	Superior and medial aspect of greater trochanter	Lateral rotation of the hip when extended (in standing). Abduction of hip when flexed	Ventral rami of S1, S2

leg areas relieved pain, and a return to fully functioning professional, family and recreational life was achieved. Therefore, the authors suggested, massage can be an effective method of reducing pain in the case of piriformis syndrome and an alternative form of conservative treatment.

Treatment Options for Piriformis Syndrome

Apply initial effleurage techniques to warm the area before beginning work over the gluteal region. As this is a very painful and sensitive area, continually gain athlete feedback; for example, use a 1–10 pain scale. Once the piriformis muscle is located, apply direct pressure for 10–30 seconds (depending on how the muscle relaxes under pressure, and the pain tolerance level of the athlete). A broader surface (like the fist) may be used initially before progressing to the (re-enforced) thumb or elbow. During the compression, check with the athlete they are not experiencing any neurological symptoms. If this does happen always decrease the pressure and/or change location. Following this, additional techniques could include deep longitudinal stripping with the knuckles, fist, forearm or fingertips from the sacrum towards the trochanter. Soft tissue release techniques should also be considered. Muscle energy techniques and the use of a myofascial release ball (tennis ball) could also be used. As with any other injury, the therapist is reminded to operate within their scope of practice and to refer the athlete to the appropriate care provider when necessary.

Neurodynamic techniques or neural tension manoeuvres are often used to assess the mobility and sensitivity of neural tissue and to determine altered nerve mechano-sensitivity. Research has indicated the mechano-sensitivity of the neural structures in the posterior leg, thigh, buttock and vertebral canal may play a part in determining the extensibility of the hamstring muscles (Castellote-Caballero et al., 2014). In this particular study, the authors found their neurodynamic sliding intervention increased short-term hamstring extensibility, measured by the passive straight leg raise (SLR), to a greater degree than static hamstring stretching. In agreement, McHugh et al. (2012) noted adverse neural tension may be a contributing factor in the high recurrence of hamstring strains (as an indicator of adhesions within the muscle or as a source of recurrent pain), and neural tension during passive stretching might be the neural mechanism for stretch-induced strength loss. For example, the authors noted, resistance to stretch was 14–15% higher for the neural tension stretch vs the neutral stretch ($p < 0.001$) at common joint angles in the final third of ROM. The authors concluded that an increased passive resistance to stretch with the addition of neural tension during passive hamstring stretch, despite no change in the EMG response, indicates passive extensibility of neural tissues can limit hamstring flexibility.

The effectiveness of treatments involving soft tissue techniques and/or neural mobilisation techniques in the management of tension-type headaches was studied by Ferragut-Garcías et al. (2017). Ninety-seven participants received either superficial massage (placebo), soft tissue techniques or a combination of soft tissue and neural mobilisation techniques. The soft tissue techniques, neural mobilisations and the combined group all improved pressure pain scores compared to baseline and placebo scores ($p < 0.001$ for all cases), but the combined group proved to be the most productive in reducing pain. And finally, twenty clinically controlled trials were included in a meta-analysis by Su and Lim (2016), comparing minimal intervention with neural mobilization on superior pain relief. This study revealed neural tissue management is superior to minimal intervention for pain relief and reduction of disability in nerve-related chronic musculoskeletal pain, although the authors concluded that their study does not establish whether it is superior to other frequently used modalities.

Special Tests

The pain elicited by the slump test is thought to be due to excessive nerve stretch (intra-neural) or reduced neural mobility at the interface with the surrounding muscle tissue (extra-neural). The athlete sits upright with their hands held together behind their back. The therapist instructs the athlete to flex their spine (slump), followed by neck flexion. The therapist then places their hand on top of the athlete's head, and the athlete then performs knee extension and dorsiflexion of the foot. Finally, the athlete returns the neck to the neutral position. The test is considered positive if symptoms are increased in the slumped position and decreased as the athlete moves out of neck flexion: sensitivity 70%, specificity 58%, positive predictive value 78%, negative predictive value 46% (Abbe et al., 2015).

The straight leg-raise (SLR) (Lasègue's sign/test or Lazarević's sign) is used to determine whether an athlete has an underlying herniated disc, often located at L5 (fifth lumbar spinal nerve). As Homayouni et al.'s (2018) study revealed, a positive SLR test for diagnosing a lumbosacral radiculopathy provides a sensitivity of 63.46% and specificity of 45.88%. Many physical tests have been described, but the accuracy of these tests and the symptoms cannot be concluded from studies to date (Hopayian & Danielyan, 2018).

The flexion, adduction, internal rotation (FAIR) test is done by examining the athlete in a seated or side-lying position. The athlete is asked to flex the hip to 90 degrees and move it along the midline. At the same time, the therapist should rotate the lower leg medially – this manoeuvre will apply tension to the piriformis muscle. Palpation will reveal tenderness over the muscle belly that stretches from the sacrum to the greater trochanter of the femur (Hicks & Varacallo, 2017).

Upper and Lower Crossed Syndrome (Pelvic Crossed Syndrome)

Upper crossed syndrome is a common postural dysfunctional movement pattern that describes the dysfunctional tone of the musculature with associated postural deviations. Janda and Jull (1987) identified two groups of muscles based on their phylogenetic development, classifying them as 'tonic' or 'phasic'. They noted the tonic system muscles are prone to tightness or shortness, and the phasic system muscles are prone to weakness or inhibition, highlighting that in addition to neurological predisposition to tightness or weakness, structural changes within the muscle also contribute to muscle imbalances. In a study of 40 patients with upper crossed syndrome (UCS) who were randomised into a treatment, the clinical efficacies of electro-acupuncture, muscle energy technique (MET) and a control group were compared following one treatment a day for 3 weeks. This study revealed that electroacupuncture plus MET can improve the pain, depression, sleep disorder, and the quality of life of UCS patients (Hua et al., 2017).

Lower crossed syndrome is characterised by tightness in the thoraco-lumbar extensors, rectus femoris and iliopsoas, as well as inhibition/weakness of the abdominals (particularly transversus abdominus) and gluteal muscles. The syndrome can lead to joint dysfunction (L4–5 and L5–S1, sacroiliac and hip joint) caused as a result of an autonomic reflex inhibition by the brain, and has shown to be a potential cause of chronic low back pain (Kim et al., 2014). Athletes will usually present with an anterior pelvic tilt, increased lumbar lordosis, lateral leg rotation and knee hyperextension (genu recurvatum). Similar to upper crossed syndrome, if massage and fascial release techniques are used in conjunction with stretching, strengthening of weaker/inhibited muscles, monitoring of training load and correct techniques, pain will reduce, and normal functional use will resume.

The anterior oblique sling is described by Chek (1998) as including the adductors of the hip, the internal oblique of the same side, the external oblique of the opposite side, the external intercostals and the pectoral group of the opposite side. He also described the posterior oblique sling as including the gluteus maximus of one side and the latissimus dorsi of the other side, joining together over the midline via the superior lamina of the posterior layer of the thoracolumbar fascia. These myofascial slings form part of Janda's muscle imbalance syndrome philosophy.

Muscles of the human body do not function as independent units. Instead, they are regarded as part of a tensegrity-like, body-wide network, with fascial structures acting as linking components. For example, it has been suggested the superficial back line is formed by the biceps femoris and erector spinae muscles, linked by the sacro-tuberous ligament and lumbar fascia (Wilke et al., 2016). Here the authors systematically reviewed 62 articles (on cadaveric dissection studies) to ascertain the scientific evidence about myofascial chains. Their review suggested most skeletal muscles of the human body are directly linked by connective tissue, but the scientific basis for the proposed connections is still a matter for debate.

Cervicogenic Headaches (CGHs)

Patients who have sustained whiplash or concussion injuries with resulting neck pain may present with cervicogenic headaches. This led Stovner et al. (2009) to suggest that headaches developing three months or more following a concussion are generally not caused by brain or head injury. Cervicogenic headaches are associated with musculoskeletal dysfunction and muscle imbalance with characteristic patterns of muscle weakness and tightness (Page, 2011), and patients with CGH often present with tightness of the sternocleidomastoid, upper trapezius, levator, scalenes, suboccipitals, pectoralis minor and pectoralis major (Zito et al., 2006). Therefore, massage and fascial release techniques applied to these areas are likely to improve symptoms.

Treatment Options for Cervicogenic Headaches

Following effleurage to the upper trapezius and neck muscles, petrissage can be used by gently lifting and picking up the tissues (Figure 9.5a) and by manipulating the musculature in a rolling fashion using the thumbs (Figure 9.5b). Deep stroking using the thumbs (Figure 9.5c) can also be used along the length of the muscle. These techniques can be repeated as necessary.

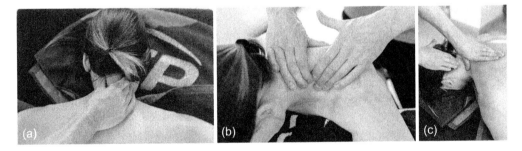

Figure 9.5 (a) Gently lift and pick up the tissues (b) thumb rolling to the upper trapezius (c) deep stroking towards the acromium process.

References

Abbe, M., Chala, M., Kebede, A., Zeleke, B. and Woldehawariat, T., 2015. Can we use seated slump test as diagnostic tool for predicting disc herniation in patients with low back pain? *Physiotherapy*, *101*, p. e27.

Barwick, A., Smith, J. and Chuter, V., 2012. The relationship between foot motion and lumbopelvic–hip function: A review of the literature. *The Foot*, *22*(3), pp. 224–231.

Brosseau, L., Wells, G.A., Poitras, S., Tugwell, P., Casimiro, L., Novikov, M., Loew, L., Sredic, D., Clément, S., Gravelle, A. and Kresic, D., 2012. Ottawa Panel evidence-based clinical practice guidelines on therapeutic massage for low back pain. *Journal of Bodywork and Movement Therapies*, 16(4), pp. 424–455.

Castellote-Caballero, Y., Valenza, M.C., Puentedura, E.J., Fernández-de-las-Peñas, C. and Alburquerque-Sendín, F., 2014. Immediate effects of neurodynamic sliding versus muscle stretching on hamstring flexibility in subjects with short hamstring syndrome. *Journal of Sports Medicine*, 2014, p. 127471. https://doi.org/10.1155/2014/127471

Chek, P., 1998. *Scientific core conditioning.* Correspondence Course, CHEK Institute, 2013.

Chun, S.W., Lim, C.Y., Kim, K., Hwang, J. and Chung, S.G., 2017. The relationships between low back pain and lumbar lordosis: A systematic review and meta-analysis. *The Spine Journal*, 17(8), pp. 1180–1191.

Daneau, C., Cantin, V. and Descarreaux, M., 2019. Effect of massage on clinical and physiological variables during muscle fatigue task in participants with chronic low back pain: A crossover study. *Journal of Manipulative and Physiological Therapeutics*, 42(1), pp. 55–65.

Elder, W.G., Munk, N., Love, M.M., Bruckner, G.G., Stewart, K.E. and Pearce, K., 2017. Real-world massage therapy produces meaningful effectiveness signal for primary care patients with chronic low back pain: Results of a repeated measures cohort study. *Pain Medicine*, 18(7), pp. 1394–1405.

Ferragut-Garcías, A., Plaza-Manzano, G., Rodríguez-Blanco, C., Velasco-Roldán, O., Pecos-Martín, D., Oliva-Pascual-Vaca, J., Llabrés-Bennasar, B. and Oliva-Pascual-Vaca, Á., 2017. Effectiveness of a treatment involving soft tissue techniques and/or neural mobilization techniques in the management of tension-type headache: A randomized controlled trial. *Archives of Physical Medicine and Rehabilitation*, 98(2), pp. 211–219.

Frenkel, M.B., Frey, C.D., Renfrow, J.J., Wolfe, S.Q., Powers, A.K. and Branch, C.L., 2018. A call for consistent radiographic definition of lumbar lordosis. *Journal of Neurosurgery: Spine*, 29(2), pp. 231–234.

Furlan, A.D., Giraldo, M., Baskwill, A., Irvin, E. and Imamura, M., 2015. Massage for low-back pain. *Cochrane Database of Systematic Reviews*, (9), CD001929. https://doi.org/10.1002/1 4651858.CD001929.pub3

Grabara, M., 2015. Comparison of posture among adolescent male volleyball players and non-athletes. *Biology of Sport*, 32(1), p. 79.

Hay, O., Dar, G., Abbas, J., Stein, D., May, H., Masharawi, Y., Peled, N. and Hershkovitz, I., 2015. The lumbar lordosis in males and females, revisited. *PLoS One*, 10(8), p. e0133685.

Hernandez-Reif, M., Field, T., Krasnegor, J. and Theakston, H., 2001. Lower back pain is reduced, and range of motion increased after massage therapy. *International Journal of Neuroscience*, 106(3–4), pp. 131–145.

Hicks, B.L. and Varacallo, M., 2017. Piriformis syndrome. In *StatPearls*. Treasure Island, FL: StatPearls Publishing.

Homayouni, K., Jafari, S.H. and Yari, H., 2018. Sensitivity and specificity of modified bragard test in patients with lumbosacral radiculopathy using electrodiagnosis as a reference standard. *Journal of Chiropractic Medicine*, 17(1), pp. 36–43.

Hopayian, K. and Danielyan, A., 2018. Four symptoms define the piriformis syndrome: An updated systematic review of its clinical features. *European Journal of Orthopaedic Surgery & Traumatology*, 28(2), pp. 155–164.

Hua, J., Shi, J. and Shen, A., 2017. Therapeutic observation of electroacupuncture plus muscle energy technique for upper crossed syndrome. *Shanghai Journal of Acupuncture and Moxibustion*, 36(1), pp. 81–84.

Janda, V. and Jull, G.A., 1987. Muscles and motor control in low back pain: Assessment and management. In T. Twomey (ed.), *Physical therapy of the low back* (pp. 253–278). New York: Churchill Livingstone.

Jandrić, S.D., 2015. Scoliosis and sport. *SportLogia*, 11(1), pp. 1–10.

Jankovic, D., Peng, P. and van Zundert, A., 2013. Brief review: Piriformis syndrome: etiology, diagnosis, and management. *Canadian Journal of Anesthesia/Journal canadien d'anesthésie*, *60*(10), pp. 1003–1012.

Joseph, L.H., Hancharoenkul, B., Sitilertpisan, P., Pirunsan, U. and Paungmali, A., 2018. Effects of massage as a combination therapy with Lumbopelvic stability exercises as compared to standard massage therapy in low Back pain: A randomized cross-over study. *International Journal of Therapeutic Massage & Bodywork*, *11*(4), p. 16.

Kim, H.J., Chung, S., Kim, S., Shin, H., Lee, J., Kim, S. and Song, M.Y., 2006. Influences of trunk muscles on lumbar lordosis and sacral angle. *European Spine Journal*, *15*(4), pp. 409–414.

Kim, J.W., Kang, M.H. and Oh, J.S., 2014. Patients with low back pain demonstrate increased activity of the posterior oblique sling muscle during prone hip extension. *PM&R*, *6*(5), pp. 400–405.

Kumar, S., Beaton, K. and Hughes, T., 2013. The effectiveness of massage therapy for the treatment of nonspecific low back pain: A systematic review of systematic reviews. *International Journal of General Medicine*, *6*, p. 733.

Lv, P., Peng, Y., Zhang, Y., Ding, K. and Chen, X., 2016. Kinematic causes and exercise rehabilitations of patients with round shoulder, thoracic kyphosis and forward head posture (FHP). *Epidemiology (Sunnyvale)*, *6*(263), pp. 2161–1165.

McHugh, M.P., Johnson, C.D. and Morrison, R.H., 2012. The role of neural tension in hamstring flexibility. *Scandinavian Journal of Medicine & Science in Sports*, *22*(2), pp. 164–169.

Page, P., 2011. Cervicogenic headaches: an evidence-led approach to clinical management. *International Journal of Sports Physical Therapy*, *6*(3), p. 254.

Purnama, M.S., Doewes, M. and Purnama, S.K., 2018. Comparison of scoliosis posture athlete's table tennis and tennis at children and adolescents. *Journal of Education, Health and Sport*, *8*(10), pp. 149–162.

Rajabi, R., Mobarakabadi, L., Alizadhen, H.M. and Hendrick, P., 2012. Thoracic kyphosis comparisons in adolescent female competitive field hockey players and untrained controls. *The Journal of Sports Medicine and Physical Fitness*, *52*(5), pp. 545–550.

Sadler, S.G., Spink, M.J., Ho, A., De Jonge, X.J. and Chuter, V.H., 2017. Restriction in lateral bending range of motion, lumbar lordosis, and hamstring flexibility predicts the development of low back pain: A systematic review of prospective cohort studies. *BMC Musculoskeletal Disorders*, *18*(1), p. 179.

Sahrmann, S.A., 2002. Movement impairment syndromes of the lumbar spine. *Diagnosis and Treatment of Movement Impairment Syndromes*, *1*, pp. 5–118.

Singla, D. and Veqar, Z., 2017. Association between forward head, rounded shoulders, and increased thoracic kyphosis: A review of the literature. *Journal of Chiropractic Medicine*, *16*(3), pp. 220–229.

Sorensen, C.J., Norton, B.J., Callaghan, J.P., Hwang, C.T. and Van Dillen, L.R., 2015. Is lumbar lordosis related to low back pain development during prolonged standing? *Manual Therapy*, *20*(4), pp. 553–557.

Stovner, L.J., Schrader, H., Mickevičiene, D., Surkiene, D. and Sand, T., 2009. Headache after concussion. *European Journal of Neurology*, *16*(1), pp. 112–120.

Su, Y. and Lim, E.C.W., 2016. Does evidence support the use of neural tissue management to reduce pain and disability in nerve-related chronic musculoskeletal pain? *The Clinical Journal of Pain*, *32*(11), pp. 991–1004.

Tchorowska, E. and Wilk, I., 2020. Application of therapeutic massage in the case of piriformis syndrome: A case study. *Pielęgniarstwo i Zdrowie Publiczne Nursing and Public Health*, *10*(2), pp. 139–144.

Thompson, T., Dias, S., Poulter, D., Weldon, S., Marsh, L., Rossato, C., Shin, J.I., Firth, J., Veronese, N., Dragioti, E. and Stubbs, B., 2020. Efficacy and acceptability of pharmacological and non-pharmacological interventions for non-specific chronic low back pain: a protocol for a systematic review and network meta-analysis. *Systematic Reviews*, *9*(1), pp. 1–11.

Wilke, J., Krause, F., Vogt, L. and Banzer, W., 2016. What is evidence-based about myofascial chains: A systematic review. *Archives of Physical Medicine and Rehabilitation*, 97(3), pp. 454–461.

Younus, A. and Kelly, A., 2020. A minimally invasive open surgical approach for piriformis syndrome. A case report and literature review. *Interdisciplinary Neurosurgery*, p. 100720.

Zito, G., Jull, G. and Story, I., 2006. Clinical tests of musculoskeletal dysfunction in the diagnosis of cervicogenic headache. *Manual Therapy*, 11(2), pp. 118–129.

10 Knowing the Sport

Tennis

Elite tennis, shown in Figure 10.1, is considered a low-risk sporting activity which requires repetitive stopping, starting, pivoting, twisting and flexion motions throughout the lower extremities, on different playing surfaces. Musculotendinous lesions are the most common type of injury (66.66%) with the incidence of lower-limb injuries higher than upper-limb and trunk lesions (Maquirriain & Baglione, 2016). Therefore, as a prevention and recovery strategy, it is

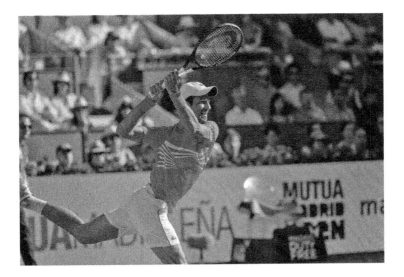

Figure 10.1 Novak Đoković, Serbian tennis player, participating in the Madrid Tennis Open.

important for the sports massage therapist to understand the biomechanics of the sport, and to assist in the prevention of muscle overload/imbalance of repetitive use and traumatic musculoskeletal injuries when they occur. The most common overuse tennis-related injuries include internal impingement and superior labrum anterior-to-posterior (SLAP) tears in the shoulder, tendinopathy at the medial or lateral elbow, tendinitis and subluxation of the extensor carpi ulnaris (ECU) tendon at the wrist, abdominal muscle strains, lumbar strains and disc degenerative pathologies (Dines et al., 2015).

DOI: 10.4324/9781003104803-10

Analysis from five years of data collection by the Association of Tennis Professionals (ATP) world tour indicated the location of overuse in the elbow, or humeral epicondyle, occurs at a 3:1 ratio (medial to lateral). It is likely that this is due to the predominance of forehand groundstrokes and serve loading in the modern game, as well as high repetitive loads that stress the medial flexor-pronator region during the acceleration phases of the serve and forehand (Kovacs & Ellenbecker, 2011). As mentioned above, injuries to the wrist are most commonly experienced as ulnar pathology relating to the extensor carpi ulnaris tendon and occur during forehand groundstrokes. The injury risk to both the ECU tendon and its fibro-osseous sheath increases when the tendon is overloaded by strong forces transmitted to the wrist at impact. In junior tennis players, playing more than 6h/week, a previous injury to the back and a previous injury regardless of location was found to be a risk factor for back pain have all been identified as risk factors for back pain (Hjelm et al., 2012). Therefore, from a therapeutic standpoint, the areas mentioned above should be addressed during therapy sessions, particularly the quadratus lumborum which get shortened on the non-dominant side.

Tennis is an asymmetrical sport even at prepubertal age. This was highlighted in a study by Sanchis-Moysi et al. (2016) who investigated the asymmetry of the pectoralis muscles in male prepubertal and adult professional tennis players. The degree of side-to-side asymmetry in pectoralis major volume was greater in prepubertal age players compared to professional players ($p < 0.05$). From a clinical perspective, this highlights the need for massage and stretching to the pectoral region on the dominant side from an early age.

Playing surface could also provide an extra injury risk; for example, during the switch from clay to the grass court season, players have to adjust to the new surface with very little preparation time. On clay there is a high and relatively gentle bounce which slows down the ball as it picks up bits of clay or moisture and becomes heavier (Martin & Prioux, 2016), whereas on grass the ball has a lower vertical bounce which means players have less time to get to the ball, and they have to stay lower. This places additional stress on the gluteal, quadricep and lower back areas. In tennis, and in all gripping-based sports, the hypothenar eminence (from lateral to medial; opponens digiti minimi, flexor digiti minimi brevis and abductor digiti minimi) and the thenar eminence (opponens pollicis, abductor pollicis brevis and the flexor pollicis brevis) can become very tight, therefore extra attention should be paid to these areas. Treatment is shown in Figures 10.2a and 10.2b.

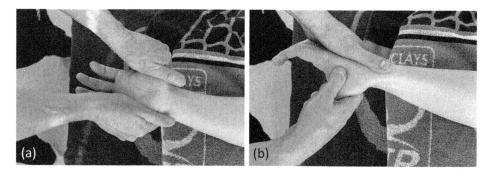

Figure 10.2 (a) Holding the athlete's hand, use the medial borders of the thumb to 'spread' the palmer surface of the hand open. Repeat 3–5 times. (b) Either small circular frictions or trigger point therapy can be used on flexor pollicis brevis and abductor pollicis brevis.

Golf

Golf (shown in Figure 10.3) is considered a low-impact sport, resulting in the common perception that only low loads and stresses are placed upon the body, and players are subjected to only a minor risk of injury (Baker et al., 2017), with most injuries occurring as a result of overuse and poor swing mechanics. Injuries to the knee are thought to account for 3–18% of all injuries in golf, with the lead knee appearing to be exposed to higher magnitudes of stress and more complex kinematics than the trailing knee (Baker et al., 2017). Other common sites of injury for males include the lower back (25–36%), followed by the left wrist (18–28%) (Lindsay & Vandervoort, 2014). In a study by McHardy et al. (2007) including 1,634 golfers, 288 reported having had one or more golf-related injuries in the previous year. The most common injury location was the lower back (25.3%), followed by the elbow (15.3%) and shoulder (9.4%). The most common injury mechanism was poor technique in the execution of the golf swing (44.8%).

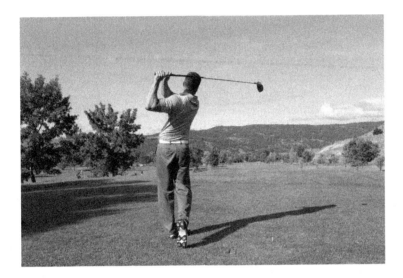

Figure 10.3 Golfer hitting a driver from the tee-box.

The modern golf swing is an asymmetrical movement that places an emphasis on restricting pelvic turn while increasing thorax rotation during the backswing to generate higher clubhead speeds at impact. Increasing thorax rotation relative to pelvic rotation preloads the trunk muscles by accentuating their length and allowing them to use the energy stored in their elastic elements to produce more power (Cole & Grimshaw, 2016). As with tennis, the asymmetry in golf and the excessive amounts of rotation, coupled with repetitive movements make corrective exercise, massage and stretching key components in keeping players injury-free.

Football

Football is one of the world's most played and watched sports across all ages and abilities (Figure 10.4), with musculoskeletal injuries occurring at every level, from grassroots to multi-million-pound professional players. Findings from a study by Blanch and Gabbett (2016) demonstrated a strong predictive (R^2 = 0.53) polynomial relationship between acute: chronic workload ratio and injury. This highlights the fact that workload and recovery principles need to be addressed, which is presumably why the majority of professional and semi-professional football clubs now have sports massage therapists to assist in the recovery process. In addition, it has been suggested that age, height, previous injuries, preferred kicking leg, impaired range of motion, muscle strength and endurance as well as poor running performance, player position, years of playing and foul play are injury risk factors in football (Stubbe et al., 2015; Svensson et al., 2016).

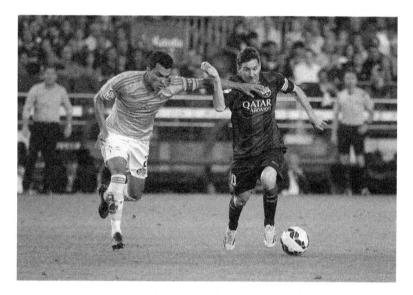

Figure 10.4 Lionel Messi (R) of FCB in action at Spanish League match between FC Barcelona and Celta de Vigo (final score 0–1) on 1 November 2014 in Camp Nou stadium, Barcelona, Spain.

More than 30% of the total number of football-related injuries consist of lower extremity muscle injuries (Stubbe et al., 2015). The occurrence of such injuries is significantly lower in matches preceded by 6 days' break (rate ratio [RR] 0.79; 95% confidence interval [CI] 0.65–0.95) or 7–10 days' break (RR 0.81; 95% CI 0.71–0.93) between matches, compared with ≤ 3 days since the last match exposure (Bengtsson et al., 2018). The hamstring muscle is the most commonly injured muscle in professional football, accounting for 37% of all muscle injuries (Ekstrand et al., 2011) with the incidence increasing by 4% per year at the Champions League level over the last decade (van Dyk et al., 2017). The dominant leg is most commonly affected in 53% (n = 56) of cases (Svensson et al., 2018). Treatment is shown in Figure 10.5.

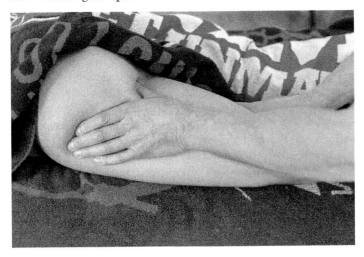

Figure 10.5 Following effleurage and petrissage techniques, deep stroking using the hand or thumb should be used, making sure techniques cover all the hamstring muscle to the attachment point (ischial tuberosity).

Cricket

Different forms of professional cricket (Test, 1 day, T20) are played in over 105 countries around the world, making it a globally played and watched sport (Figure 10.6). The majority of injuries are of a non-contact nature and have traditionally been thought of as 'overuse' injuries (Orchard et al., 2016). The incidence of injuries within cricket remains high: a study among English players found 23% of players sustained a shoulder injury during a single season, with the majority affected in the throwing arm (Ranson & Gregory, 2008). Lower limb injuries form nearly 49.8% of injuries, followed by back injuries (22.8%), upper limb injuries (23.3%)

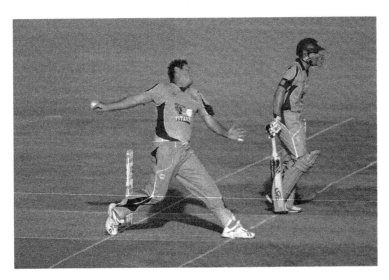

Figure 10.6 Action during a one-day cricket match between the Eagles and Titans (Titans won by four wickets) on 22 December 2009 in Bloemfontein, South Africa.

and neck injuries (4.1%). Other common injuries include lateral epicondylitis (tennis elbow), which is common in batsmen and is often caused by improper batting biomechanics or inappropriate equipment such as a heavy bat (Pardiwala et al., 2018). As in professional football, the most common (highest incidence) injury over a decade was hamstring strains (8.7 match time-loss injuries per 100 players per year). Other prevalent injuries are lumbar stress fractures, causing 1.9% of players to be unavailable, which represents 15% of all missed playing time (Orchard et al., 2016). In the quadricep muscle group the rectus femoris is the most frequently injured component, and the strain is classically at the distal musculotendinous junction, midportion or the proximal insertion (Pardiwala et al., 2018).

Rugby

Rugby (union), shown in Figure 10.7, is classed as a contact or collision sport and is played in the northern and southern hemispheres, in both 15- and 7-a-side formats. Unsurprisingly, injury rates have shown to be as high as 57.2 per 1,000 player-hours, with most injuries being muscular and player position not influencing the injury rate and type (Azman et al., 2016).

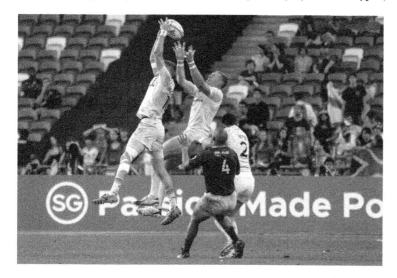

Figure 10.7 England 7s team playing against South Africa 7s team during Day 2 of HSBC World Rugby Singapore Sevens on 29 April 2018 at National Stadium in Singapore.

The results of a meta-analysis by Yeomans et al. (2018) confirmed the match injury incidence rate of 46.8/1,000 player-hours in amateur rugby is low in comparison with professional cohorts, with a pooled incidence rate of 81/1,000 player-hours (95% CI 34.4–59.2). The results of this meta-analysis showed the tackle event, specifically injuries to the tackler, accounted for the highest incidence of injury (15.9/1,000 player-hours; 95% CI 12.4–19). This is probably a result of professional players being quicker and heavier and playing on better pitches than their amateur counterparts.

The strongest predictors for lower extremity injuries in rugby union players are uneven hips, pronated feet, tight hamstrings, anatomical leg length differences, gait pronation, tall stature and certain postural and biomechanical imbalances in the lower extremities (Bruwer et al., 2017). Aside from general recovery massage, it would be advisable to work on areas where imbalances have occurred, and in the hamstrings and gastrocnemius area.

Swimming

Swimming, shown in Figure 10.8, can be recreational, rehabilitation or a highly competitive sport requiring high levels of training and performance which can cause overuse of the musculoskeletal system, leading to injuries (Adiele & Morgan, 2018). The majority of these injuries are caused by poor stroke biomechanics, overuse and fatigue of the shoulder muscles, scapula and upper back, and glenohumeral laxity with subsequent shoulder instability (Butler et al., 2015; de Almeida et al., 2015). Freestyle, butterfly, backstroke and breaststroke are the four strokes for competitive swimming events, and all involve a repetitive motion. Backstroke swimmers have more shoulder injuries than other strokes, as the backstroke forces humeral internal rotation sprain in the upper limb elevation during the catching motion. The incidence of injuries is greater in female swimmers, and in swimmers of an older age (Matsuura et al., 2019).

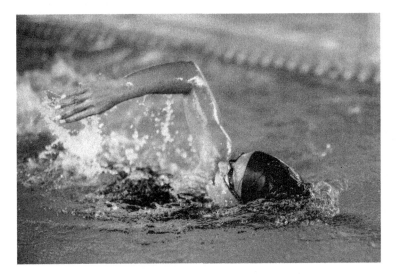

Figure 10.8 Professional swimmer during a swimming race.

It is not unreasonable to presume there is an association between swim-training volume and shoulder pain in competitive swimmers. This was corroborated by Feijen and colleagues (2020), who demonstrated that adolescent competitive swimmers as a group showed the highest prevalence of shoulder pain and a moderate level of evidence for a relationship with swim-training volume. However, the term 'swimmer's shoulder' does not define a specific clinical diagnosis, and its aetiology is considered to be multifactorial. In the literature, shoulder pain prevalence varies according to the adopted definitions from 3% to 91% (Tessaro et al., 2017). This variation could be a result of swimmers who train more and show higher pressure pain thresholds, indicating lower pain sensitivity (Kuppens et al., 2019).

With high volume training, swimming injuries can occur in other areas of the body, including the neck, lower back and knee. For example, if one considers the number of strokes a freestyle swimmer takes, i.e., up to 5,000 strokes per session, and the swimmer breathes every three strokes, they would be turning their head 1,667 times to breathe per session (Pollard & Fernandez, 2004). Swimmer's knee mostly occurs in breaststroke swimmers, but also in other swimming disciplines, and is considered to be the cause of the symptoms of enthesitis of the medial collateral ligament insertions on the medial femoral epicondyle (Kezunovic, 2013). In addition, the hyperextension motion of the lumbar spine seen with butterfly and breaststroke can predispose to facet joint irritation (Pollard & Fernandez, 2004). Due to muscle imbalances, particularly between the internal and external shoulder rotators, special attention should be paid to massage and stretching of the latissimus dorsi, deltoid, pectorals and shoulder internal rotators, which characteristically shorten. In addition, the muscles around the thoracic spine should be loosened to prevent a loss of thoracic extension.

Long-Distance Running

Participation in long-distance running events (Figure 10.9) has grown significantly in the last decade (Ogueta-Alday et al., 2018). Distance running (10k–marathon) is a strenuous activity due to the prolonged duration and eccentric component; it is therefore not without risk. Running injuries are multifactorial and involve both extrinsic and intrinsic factors, including altered running biomechanics; poor technique affecting step rate, step length and foot strike pattern (mid/fore/rear foot); running surface; age; environmental conditions; rapidly increased training load/volume; gender; previous injury and/or incorrect footwear, all of which *could* be responsible for present or future injuries.

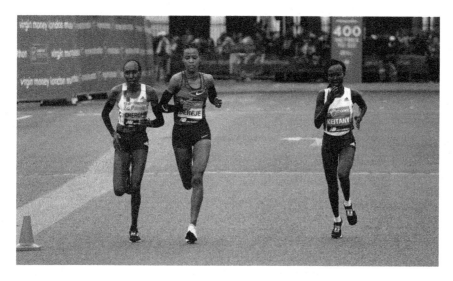

Figure 10.9 Virgin Money London Marathon 2019's elite women event, about 350 yards from the finish line.

Francis et al. (2019) conducted a systematic review investigating injury proportion by anatomical location and gender (10,688 injuries reported from 18,195 runners included in 36 reviewed studies). The authors noted that the knee (28%) and ankle-foot (26%) regions accounted for over half of all the injuries reported (n = 5,816/10,688). The third highest proportion of injury was at the shank (16%). The authors' data indicated 70% of all injuries reported were at or below the knee. The hip and thigh regions accounted for 14% of injuries. Interestingly, the authors concluded women have a larger proportion of knee injuries (40% of all injuries), relative to men, who experience a similar proportion of knee (31%) and ankle-foot (26%) injuries. This could be due to hormonal factors, a wider Q angle, poorer neuromuscular control and/or lack of quadricep and gluteal strength.

Other studies have identified common 'injury prone' areas in long distance runners. Magnan et al. (2014) cited Achilles tendinopathy and fasciopathy, plantar fasciitis, iliotibial band friction syndrome and medial tibial stress syndrome as regularly injured areas. However, they reported the most prevalent injury site is the knee, with anterior knee pain reported more often than other injuries. Lachniet et al. (2018) noted that the stress reaction afflicting distance runners is medial tibial stress syndrome (MTSS), which can progress to a tibial stress fracture if bone stress continues to exceed bone repair and healing.

Running injuries across younger and older populations have been investigated. Devita et al. (2016) found inverse and linear relations between age and basic running kinematics: as age increased, stride length and running velocity decreased. On the basis of the regression equations, the authors estimated that stride length and running velocity were reduced by 0.08 m and 0.10 m/s^{-1} over each decade. During the ageing process from 20 to 60 years of age, these equations predict that average stride length and running velocity will decrease from 2.37 to 2.05 m and from 3.23 to 2.81 m/s^{-1} (both 20%). Notably, the authors observed reduced ankle joint moment and power with age but not reduced knee or hip joint moment and power. Eighteen per cent of youth marathon participants (mean age 15) reported an injury over the course of an eight-month training program. The majority of injuries were acute. There was no significant difference in injury rates between males and females, but high school (HS) runners were more likely to be injured than middle school (MS) runners (99.6% of study participants successfully completed the marathon, a higher completion rate than seen in adults) (Goldman & Beck, 2019).

In 3,768 runners the overall risk model in short- and long-distance runners contained four risk factors: previous injuries (odds ratio [OR] 3.7) and running distance during the event (OR 1.3) increased the risk of a running injury, whereas older age (OR 0.99) and more training kilometres per week (OR 0.99) showed a decrease. Models between short and long-distance runners did not differ significantly. Previous injuries increased the risk of a running injury in all models, while more training kilometres per week decreased this risk (van Poppel et al., 2018).

Furthermore, following a half marathon, massage can be recommended for restoring subjective fatigue measures (but not objective fatigue markers). Therefore, it could provide only a psychological advantage with no clear benefits on physiological fatigue (Wiewelhove et al., 2018). As most competitive long-distance runners have days, weeks, or even months to recover, it would be advisable to concentrate massage techniques to all the lower body musculature and, if required, the lower back and thoracic area, to promote psychological and physiological recovery.

Cycling

Cycling, shown in Figure 10.10, is a popular sport that has participants of many different ages, with a wide variety of skill and fitness levels. Elite cyclists training for and participating in major events are subject to injuries (Haeberle et al., 2018). Common injuries include knee pain, patella quadriceps tendinitis, iliotibial band syndrome, stress fracture, compartment syndrome, numbness of the foot and metatarsalgia (Wanich et al., 2007).

A study conducted by De Bernardo et al. (2012) over a 4-year period examined 51 top-level cyclists. The authors found the prevalence of overuse and traumatic injuries to be nearly equal in top-level cyclists (48.5% traumatic and 51.5% overuse), with 68.5% of overuse injuries located in the lower limb. Cycling parameters (i.e., cadence and power output) and bicycle fit settings have differing effects on kinematics, kinetics and muscle activity around the knee (Johnston et al., 2017). Therefore, to increase performance and help reduce the prevalence of

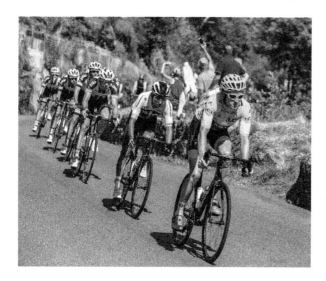

Figure 10.10 Egan Arley Bernal riding behind Geraint Thomas in the lead on a descending road in the Occitan region during the Tour de France 2018.

injury, correct bike set-up should be addressed, alongside therapeutic massage interventions, with special attention paid to the quadriceps, hip flexors, erector spinae and iliotibial band region. In addition, with the growing popularity of mountain biking, the number of riders at risk for an acute injury has increased with an equal prevalence of acute injuries in elite and amateur mountain bikers (Stoop et al., 2019), although it should be noted that some of these injuries may be of a traumatic nature, from falls.

References

Adiele, D. and Morgan, G.P., 2018. Prevalence of musculoskeletal injuries in males and females practicing swimming from higher school of Zimbabwe. *American Journal of Sports Science*, 6(1), pp. 8–11.

Azman, M.A.A.M., Lan, N.C., Azmi, S.H. and Sulaiman, N., 2016, November. A systematic review of type of injury among rugby union players. In: Sulaiman, N., Ismail, S., Adnan, R. (eds), *International colloquium on sport science, exercise, engineering and technology* (pp. 35–42). Singapore: Springer. https://doi.org/10.1007/978-981-10-6772-3_5.

Baker, M.L., Epari, D.R., Lorenzetti, S., Sayers, M., Boutellier, U. and Taylor, W.R., 2017. Risk factors for knee injury in golf: A systematic review. *Sports Medicine*, 47(12), pp. 2621–2639.

Bengtsson, H., Ekstrand, J., Waldén, M. and Hägglund, M., 2018. Muscle injury rate in professional football is higher in matches played within 5 days since the previous match: A 14-year prospective study with more than 130 000 match observations. *British Journal of Sports Medicine*, 52(17), pp. 1116–1122.

Blanch, P. and Gabbett, T.J., 2016. Has the athlete trained enough to return to play safely? The acute: Chronic workload ratio permits clinicians to quantify a player's risk of subsequent injury. *British Journal of Sports Medicine*, 50(8), pp. 471–475.

Bruwer, E.J., Moss, S.J. and Jacobs, S., 2017. Injury incidence and selected biomechanical, postural and anthropometric characteristics contributing to musculoskeletal injuries in rugby union players. *African Journal for Physical Activity and Health Sciences (AJPHES)*, 23(1.2), pp. 172–189.

Butler, D., Funk, L., Mackenzie, T.A. and Herrington, L.C., 2015. Sorting swimmers shoulders: An observational study on swimmers that presented to a shoulder surgeon. *International Journal of Shoulder Surgery*, 9(3), p. 90.

Cole, M.H. and Grimshaw, P.N., 2016. The biomechanics of the modern golf swing: Implications for lower back injuries. *Sports Medicine*, 46(3), pp. 339–351.

de Almeida, M.O., Hespanhol, L.C. and Lopes, A.D., 2015. Prevalence of musculoskeletal pain among swimmers in an elite national tournament. *International Journal of Sports Physical Therapy*, 10(7), p. 1026.

De Bernardo, N., Barrios, C., Vera, P., Laíz, C. and Hadala, M., 2012. Incidence and risk for traumatic and overuse injuries in top-level road cyclists. *Journal of Sports Sciences*, 30(10), pp. 1047–1053.

Devita, P., Fellin, R.E., Seay, J.F., Ip, E., Stavro, N. and Messier, S.P., 2016. The relationships between age and running biomechanics. *Medicine and Science in Sports and Exercise*, 48(1), pp. 98–106.

Dines, J.S., Bedi, A., Williams, P.N., Dodson, C.C., Ellenbecker, T.S., Altchek, D.W., Windler, G. and Dines, D.M., 2015. Tennis injuries: Epidemiology, pathophysiology, and treatment. *JAAOS-Journal of the American Academy of Orthopaedic Surgeons*, 23(3), pp. 181–189.

Ekstrand, J., Hägglund, M. and Waldén, M., 2011. Injury incidence and injury patterns in professional football: the UEFA injury study. *British Journal of Sports Medicine*, 45(7), pp. 553–558.

Feijen, S., Tate, A., Kuppens, K., Claes, A. and Struyf, F., 2020. Swim-Training volume and shoulder pain across the life span of the competitive swimmer: A systematic review. *Journal of Athletic Training*, 55(1), pp. 32–41.

Francis, P., Whatman, C., Sheerin, K., Hume, P. and Johnson, M.I., 2019. The proportion of lower limb running injuries by gender, anatomical location and specific pathology: A systematic review. *Journal of Sports Science & Medicine*, 18(1), p. 21.

Goldman, J. and Beck, J., 2019. Youth marathon training: Injury epidemiology & risk factors. *Orthopaedic Journal of Sports Medicine*, 7(3_suppl), p. 2325967119S00063.

Haeberle, H.S., Navarro, S.M., Power, E.J., Schickendantz, M.S., Farrow, L.D. and Ramkumar, P.N., 2018. Prevalence and epidemiology of injuries among elite cyclists in the tour de France. *Orthopaedic Journal of Sports Medicine*, 6(9), p. 2325967118793392.

Hjelm, N., Werner, S. and Renstrom, P., 2012. Injury risk factors in junior tennis players: A prospective 2-year study. *Scandinavian Journal of Medicine & Science in Sports*, 22(1), pp. 40–48.

Johnston, T.E., Baskins, T.A., Koppel, R.V., Oliver, S.A., Stieber, D.J. and Hoglund, L.T., 2017. The influence of extrinsic factors on knee biomechanics during cycling: A systematic review of the literature. *International Journal of Sports Physical Therapy*, 12(7), p. 1023.

Kezunovic, M., 2013. Overuse knee injuries in athletes. *Montenegrin Journal of Sports Science and Medicine*, 2(1), pp. 29–32.

Kovacs, M. and Ellenbecker, T., 2011. An 8-stage model for evaluating the tennis serve: implications for performance enhancement and injury prevention. *Sports Health*, 3(6), pp. 504–513.

Kuppens, K., Feijen, S., Roussel, N., Nijs, J., Cras, P., van Wilgen, P. and Struyf, F., 2019. Training volume is associated with pain sensitivity, but not with endogenous pain modulation, in competitive swimmers. *Physical Therapy in Sport*, 37, pp. 150–156.

Lachniet, P.B., Taylor-Haas, J.A., Paterno, M.V., DiCesare, C.A. and Ford, K.R., 2018. Altered sagittal plane hip biomechanics in adolescent male distance runners with a history of lower extremity injury. *International Journal of Sports Physical Therapy*, 13(3), p. 441.

Lindsay, D.M. and Vandervoort, A.A., 2014. Golf-related low back pain: A review of causative factors and prevention strategies. *Asian Journal of Sports Medicine*, 5(4), p. e24289. https://doi.org/10.5812/asjsm.24289.

Magnan, B., Bondi, M., Pierantoni, S. and Samaila, E., 2014. The pathogenesis of Achilles tendinopathy: A systematic review. *Foot and Ankle Surgery*, 20(3), pp. 154–159.

Maquirriain, J. and Baglione, R., 2016. Epidemiology of tennis injuries: An eight-year review of Davis Cup retirements. *European Journal of Sport Science*, 16(2), pp. 266–270.

Martin, C. and Prioux, J., 2016. Tennis playing surfaces: The effects on performance and injuries. *Journal of Medicine and Science in Tennis*, 21(1), pp. 11–19.

Matsuura, Y., Hangai, M., Koizumi, K., Ueno, K., Hirai, N., Akuzawa, H. and Kaneoka, K., 2019. Injury trend analysis in the Japan national swim team from 2002 to 2016: effect of the lumbar injury prevention project. *BMJ Open Sport & Exercise Medicine*, 5(1), p. e000615. doi:10.1136/bmjsem-2019-.

McHardy, A., Pollard, H. and Lou, K., 2007. The epidemiology of golf related injuries in Australian amateur golfers-a multivariate analysis. *South African Journal of Sports Medicine*, 19(1), pp. 12–19.

Ogueta-Alday, A., Morante, J.C., Gómez-Molina, J. and García-López, J., 2018. Similarities and differences among half-marathon runners according to their performance level. *PloS One*, 13(1), p. e0191688.

Orchard, J.W., Kountouris, A. and Sims, K., 2016. Incidence and prevalence of elite male cricket injuries using updated consensus definitions. *Open Access Journal of Sports Medicine*, 7, p. 187.

Pardiwala, D.N., Rao, N.N. and Varshney, A.V., 2018. Injuries in cricket. *Sports Health*, 10(3), pp. 217–222.

Pollard, H. and Fernandez, M., 2004. Spinal musculoskeletal injuries associated with swimming: a discussion of technique. *Australasian Chiropractic & Osteopathy*, 12(2), p. 72.

Ranson, C. and Gregory, P.L., 2008. Shoulder injury in professional cricketers. *Physical Therapy in Sport*, 9(1), pp. 34–39.

Sanchis-Moysi, J., Dorado, C., Idoate, F., González-Henríquez, J.J., Serrano-Sanchez, J.A. and Calbet, J.A., 2016. The asymmetry of pectoralis muscles is greater in male prepubertal than in professional tennis players. *European Journal of Sport Science*, 16(7), pp. 780–786.

Stoop, R., Hohenauer, E., Vetsch, T., Deliens, T. and Clijsen, R., 2019. Acute injuries in male elite and amateur mountain bikers: Results of a survey. *Journal of Sports Science & Medicine*, 18(2), p. 207.

Stubbe, J.H., van Beijsterveldt, A.M.M., van der Knaap, S., Stege, J., Verhagen, E.A., Van Mechelen, W. and Backx, F.J., 2015. Injuries in professional male soccer players in the Netherlands: A prospective cohort study. *Journal of Athletic Training*, 50(2), pp. 211–216.

Svensson, K., Alricsson, M., Karnebäck, G., Magounakis, T. and Werner, S., 2016. Muscle injuries of the lower extremity: A comparison between young and old male elite soccer players. *Knee Surgery, Sports Traumatology, Arthroscopy*, 24(7), pp. 2293–2299.

Svensson, K., Eckerman, M., Alricsson, M., Magounakis, T. and Werner, S., 2018. Muscle injuries of the dominant or non-dominant leg in male football players at elite level. *Knee Surgery, Sports Traumatology, Arthroscopy*, 26(3), pp. 933–937.

Tessaro, M., Granzotto, G., Poser, A., Plebani, G. and Rossi, A., 2017. Shoulder pain in competitive teenage swimmers and its prevention: a retrospective epidemiological cross-sectional study of prevalence. *International Journal of Sports Physical Therapy*, 12(5), p. 798.

van Dyk, N., Bahr, R., Burnett, A.F., Whiteley, R., Bakken, A., Mosler, A., Farooq, A. and Witvrouw, E., 2017. A comprehensive strength testing protocol offers no clinical value in predicting risk of hamstring injury: A prospective cohort study of 413 professional football players. *British Journal of Sports Medicine*, 51(23), pp. 1695–1702.

van Poppel, D., Scholten-Peeters, G.G., van Middelkoop, M., Koes, B.W. and Verhagen, A.P., 2018. Risk models for lower extremity injuries among short-and long-distance runners: A prospective cohort study. *Musculoskeletal Science and Practice*, 36, pp. 48–53.

Wanich, T., Hodgkins, C., Columbier, J.A., Muraski, E. and Kennedy, J.G., 2007. Cycling injuries of the lower extremity. *JAAOS-Journal of the American Academy of Orthopaedic Surgeons*, 15(12), pp. 748–756.

Wiewelhove, T., Schneider, C., Döwcling, A., Hanakam, F., Rasche, C., Meyer, T., Kellmann, M., Pfeiffer, M. and Ferrauti, A., 2018. Effects of different recovery strategies following a half-marathon on fatigue markers in recreational runners. *PloS One*, 13(11), p. e0207313.

Yeomans, C., Kenny, I.C., Cahalan, R., Warrington, G.D., Harrison, A.J., Hayes, K., Lyons, M., Campbell, M.J. and Comyns, T.M., 2018. The incidence of injury in amateur male rugby union: A systematic review and meta-analysis. *Sports Medicine*, 48(4), pp. 837–848.

11 Associated Treatment Modalities

Foam Rolling

Foam rollers are frequently used by amateur and professional athletes, fitness instructors, personal trainers, and massage and sports therapists in treatment rooms and gyms as part of warm up, recovery and rehabilitation routines (see Figure 11.1). However, there seems to be a lack of understanding by therapists and athletes on why and how to use them. During foam rolling, the athlete lies across a foam cylinder and uses body weight to control the pressure, then rolls the cylinder along a section of muscle, beginning distally and moving proximally. Any positive effects of self-myofascial release (SMR) using a roller could be as a result of increasing fascia's sliding properties by breaking up adhesions or loosening cross-links, as well as stimulating contractile cell activity and affecting tissue hydration with the added compression of the muscle and fascial tissue (Schleip & Muller, 2013). However, a review by Behm and Wilke (2019) noted that there is insufficient evidence to support the claim that the primary mechanisms underlying rolling and other similar devices are the release of myofascial restrictions, and thus the term 'self-myofascial release devices' is misleading.

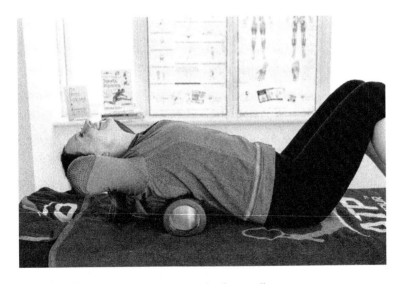

Figure 11.1 Thoracic extension over the foam roller.

DOI: 10.4324/9781003104803-11

Performance Outcomes

In a study by Healey and colleagues (2014), no significant differences were found between foam roller and planking exercises on performance measures in four athletic tests comprising vertical jump for height, vertical jump for power, isometric squat and an agility drill speed test. However, post-exercise fatigue ratings (using a Likert scale) after foam rolling was significantly less than after the subjects (n = 26) performed planking ($p \leq 0.05$). MacDonald et al. (2013) measured quadriceps' maximal voluntary contraction force (MVC) and found subjects were able to produce similar amounts of force in both the foam rolling and control conditions, indicating that foam rolling had no effect on performance. In agreement, Hodgson et al. (2018) used 23 recreationally active students over a 4-week period to roll three or six days a week (four sets of 30 seconds). Range of motion (ROM), electromyographic (EMG) activity, countermovement jump (CMJ) and maximal voluntary isometric contraction (MVIC) forces were assessed. The major findings in this study indicated roller massage training performed either three or six days per week did not improve any of the physiological or performance measures with the rolled or contralateral limbs, indicating that previously reported rolling-induced acute improvements may be transient.

An investigation by D'Amico et al. (2020) indicated that when compared to a control group, foam rolling (on both the right and left legs, for two 60-second bouts each) can reduce perceptions of muscle soreness following exercise-induced muscle damage (EIMD) caused by sprinting. Conversely, the results indicate that foam rolling does not impact recovery of agility (T-test time), enhance recovery of vertical jump (VJ), increase heart rate variability (HRV) or decrease pulse wave velocity (PWV) compared to a control group. Similarly, a study of 18 professional football players examining the effectiveness of 20 minutes of foam rolling exercises as opposed to passive rest during recovery was designed by Rey et al. (2019). The authors investigated total quality of recovery, perceived muscle soreness, jump performance, agility and flexibility. Their analysis revealed foam rolling had the greatest effect on recovery and perceived muscle soreness, compared to the passive recovery group, 24 hours after training. Peacock and colleagues (2015) investigated the use of a foam roller as part of a warm-up routine in 11 physically active athletic males, and demonstrated greater performance scores for vertical jump, standing long jump, a pro-agility test and a 1 rep max bench press when it was added to a dynamic warm-up protocol. However, in this study the foam roller did not improve flexibility in a sit and reach test. Furthermore, 14 female college athletes using a foam roller (for 6 minutes) as part of a warm-up routine indicated improvement in squat jump and countermovement jump, with no detrimental effects on flexibility, drop jump, sprint and agility performance (Rickman et al., 2019).

Lyu et al.'s (2020) study investigated the immediate effects of vibration rolling (VR) (28 Hz, 30 seconds × 3 sets on both calf muscles) combined with dynamic muscle contraction as a warm-up protocol on the ankle ROM, proprioception, muscle strength and agility. Regarding the effects on ankle ROM, both foam-rolling with dynamic muscle contraction (DVR) and VR significantly improved ankle dorsiflexion ROM and plantar flexion; in addition, DVR more significantly improved dorsiflexion ROM than VR ($p < 0.001$). The authors concluded that there is no consensus on the optimal VR technique, including vibration frequency and combination of rolling techniques (i.e., coupled with active joint motion during rolling), although from their research DVR appears to be a beneficial warm-up protocol to enhance exercise performance. In addition, Cheatham et al. (2019) compared vibration rolling to non-vibration rolling and to a non-rolling control group. The authors' data indicated that the positive results demonstrated by their vibration roller group may be due to the increase in an individual's tolerance to pain more effectively than a non-vibration roller.

Twenty-one studies were included in a comprehensive meta-analysis by Wiewelhove et al. (2019). Fourteen studies used pre-rolling, while seven studies used post-rolling. Pre-rolling resulted in a small improvement in sprint performance (+0.7%, g = 0.28) and flexibility (+4.0%, g = 0.34), whereas the effect on jump (–1.9%, g = 0.09) and strength performance (+1.8%, g = 0.12) was negligible. Post-rolling slightly attenuated exercise-induced decreases in sprint (+3.1%, g = 0.34) and strength performance (+3.9%, g = 0.21). It also reduced muscle pain perception (+6.0%, g = 0.47), whereas its effect on jump performance (–0.2%, g = 0.06) was trivial. Furthermore, in a systematic review (49 articles) by Hendricks et al. (2019), the authors reported foam rolling may reduce muscle stiffness and increase ROM and should be used in combination with dynamic stretching and active warm up before a training session. Furthermore, the optimum dosage to achieve these flexibility benefits seems to be a total of 90–120 seconds of foam rolling, which reduced delayed onset muscle soreness (DOMS) and increased pressure pain threshold (PPT) and therefore may optimise recovery from training. Finally, a recent systematic review and meta-analysis (32 studies) conducted by Skinner et al. (2020) indicated that foam rolling increases range of motion, appears to be useful for recovery from exercise-induced muscle damage, and seems to have no detrimental effect on other athletic performance measures. However, the authors added, except for range of motion, it cannot be concluded that foam rolling is directly beneficial to athletic performance.

How Long Should an Athlete Roll For?

The duration of the 'hold' in foam rolling protocols (ischemic compressions) varies, with current self-myofascial release recommendations calling for the user to hold the foam roller on an area of tense muscle for 30–90 seconds, depending on pain tolerance, or until a 'release' is felt (Schleip, 2003a; Lavelle et al., 2007). Results from 55 papers included in Dębski et al.'s (2019) review of the literature indicated that desirable forms of treatment, in terms of therapeutic effect, are treatments using a firmer type of roller, with as great a force of application as possible (as tolerated by the patient), for a period of 30–120 seconds. The intensity of a single rolling movement should be moderate, and the movement should last about 3 seconds. Keeping the roller on particularly sensitive areas is recommended. During the course of one session, it is worth using between one and three applications, separated by a 30-second break.

Blood Flow

A study by Okamoto et al. (2014) found foam rolling significantly reduced vascular stiffness and improved endothelial arterial function, providing supportive evidence to the theory that foam rolling does improve blood flow. In agreement, values were assessed (Hotfiel et al., 2017) under resting conditions, and twice after foam rolling exercises (0 and 30 minutes after the rolling intervention) in 21 healthy individuals. The trochanteric region, mid portion and distal tibial insertion of the lateral thigh were presented for the authors' data analysis. The results from this study indicated arterial blood flow of the lateral thigh increased significantly after foam rolling exercises compared with baseline ($p \leq 0.05$). Therefore, results seem to be positive on the effects of foam rolling on arterial blood flow/function, although this area needs to be researched more thoroughly before firm conclusions can be drawn.

Range of Motion

The majority of studies on self-myofascial release with a foam roller have investigated flexibility and range of motion, including MacDonald et al. (2013). The authors indicated there was a significant increase in knee joint ROM at 2 minutes post-foam rolling (12.7%) and 10 minutes post-foam rolling (10.3%) of the quadriceps muscles. Results highlighted no significant changes in voluntary or evoked muscle properties after foam rolling, and after foam rolling the negative correlation between ROM and force production no longer existed. This led the researchers to conclude that the high force mechanical stress application (i.e. a combination of body mass and high-pressure foam rolling) performed in their study was enough to induce a gel-like state in the fascia, leading to increased soft tissue compliance and subsequently greater knee joint ROM.

Roylance and colleagues (2013) found an acute treatment of foam rolling with postural alignment exercises and/or static stretches significantly increased range of motion (sit and reach test) in participants with below average flexibility. Also using the sit and reach test to assess flexibility, Paz et al. (2017) found no improvements using a foam roller compared to a traditional cycle warm up when foam rolling was performed on both limbs in an alternating manner, adopting 30 seconds for each leg (knee flexor and triceps surae muscles). Jay et al. (2014), again using the sit and reach test, found a short-term increase in flexibility, but unfortunately these gains appeared to last for only 10 minutes. Both foam rolling and roller massager increased hip flexion and hip extension in 18 recreationally resistance-trained males (Monteiro et al., 2018), although once again the effects were short-lived, with the authors noting increases in range of motion starting to fall in as little as 10 minutes. Similarly, positive effects lasting less than 10 minutes were also noted by Skarabot et al. (2015) when foam rolling and static stretching were combined (compared to foam rolling alone), suggesting it may be important to study the time course effects of foam rolling. Additionally, positive short-term effects of foam rolling were also noted by Kelly and Beardsley (2016). The authors found improvements in ankle dorsiflexion range of motion for at least 20 minutes in the ipsilateral limb and up to 10 minutes in the contralateral limb, indicating that foam rolling produces a cross-over effect into the contralateral limb. The mechanism producing these cross-over effects are unclear but may involve increased stretch tolerance, as observed following static stretching.

Madoni et al. (2018) examined the effects of foam rolling on range of motion, peak torque, muscle activation and hamstring to quadricep (H:Q) strength ratios in 22 recreationally active women. The results from this study led the authors to conclude that foam rolling produces greater changes in hamstring ROM than other methods of stretching or a control group, without creating a deficit in peak torque or muscle activation. Therefore, foam rolling may be beneficial in increasing ROM without decreasing functional H:Q ratios.

Seventeen recreationally active students took part in a study by Sullivan and associates in 2013, examining the effects of short duration foam rolling (5–10 seconds) on the sit and reach test and in neuromuscular activity, via EMG (in the hamstrings). A 4.3% increase in sit and reach scores after 5 seconds was noted, with a greater trend of increased ROM after 10 seconds, although there were no changes in EMG activity. Interestingly in this piece of research the authors added 13 kg of additional weights to vertical poles as a rolling device. In addition, Junker and Stoggl (2015) compared foam rolling to contract-relax (PNF) stretching in 40 volunteers, with both groups showing improvements in hamstring flexibility compared to their control group. In 2014, Mohr et al. investigated foam rolling prior to static stretching in 40 subjects over six treatment sessions and found a greater increase in hip flexion ROM compared to the static stretching group, although a shorter duration of up to 2 minutes did not improve knee joint flexibility. By contrast, Halperin et al. (2014), following three sets of 30 seconds with 10 seconds of inter-set rest, found both roller massage and static stretching significantly increased ankle range of motion, although there was no difference between the interventions. Su et al. (2017) concluded that foam rolling is more effective than static and dynamic stretching in acutely increasing flexibility of the quadriceps and hamstrings without hampering muscle strength, and may be recommended as part of a warm up in healthy young adults. Increases in range of motion were also noted in another study using foam rollers compared to a roller massager (Monteiro et al., 2019). The authors concluded that both the foam roller and roller massager increased hip range of motion, with the foam roller producing the greatest increases.

In addition, in subjects consisting of NCAA Division 1 offensive linesmen, hip flexibility was statistically significantly increased when tested after both dynamic stretching and foam rolling ($p = 0.0001$), although no changes in strength or power were evident. The authors suggested that increased flexibility after deep tissue rolling may be used interchangeably with traditional stretching exercises (Behara & Jacobson, 2017). A modified Thomas Test was used to assess the effects of foam rolling on knee flexion ROM and rectus femoris length in 23 participants (Vigotski et al., 2015). The authors found no significant improvements following two 1-minute bouts of foam rolling, although they believed this could have been due to the type and length of warm up selected prior to rolling. Taking into account rolling duration, Couture et al. (2015) also showed no significant differences between baseline knee extension ROM and the ROM present after foam rolling, for either a short (two sets of 10 seconds) or long (four sets of 30 seconds) duration. Finally, in a recent systematic review and multi-level meta-analysis (26 trials with high methodological quality), Wilke et al. (2020) revealed that foam rolling (with or without vibration) represents an effective method to induce acute improvements in joint ROM. In summary, any short- or longer-lasting improvement in range of motion from foam rolling could be useful for a competing athlete, particularly as it appears from the literature that there is unlikely to be a loss in performance outcomes.

Delayed Onset Muscle Soreness

The use of foam rollers in the recovery from delayed onset muscle soreness has been investigated (MacDonald, 2013) with some positive results. Following ten sets of ten repetitions of squats at 60% max, 20 physically active males received two bouts of 60-second foam rolling per exercise at 0, 24 and 48 hours. The authors found that foam rolling using 26–46 kg (32–55% of subjects' body weight) produced significant reduction from DOMS at 24, 48 and 72 hours post-workout, and improved vertical jump height. In agreement, Jay et al. (2014) investigated the acute effect of massage with a roller massager on hamstring muscle soreness directly in one leg, and also any potential cross-over effects to the non-massaged leg, in 22 volunteers. All participants performed ten sets of ten repetitions of stiff-legged deadlifts with a kettlebell, separated by 30 seconds of rest at a speed of 1–2 seconds for the concentric and eccentric phases of each repetition. Measurements of soreness, pressure pain threshold and flexibility were taken before and at 0, 10, 30 and 60 minutes post-foam rolling treatment. The researchers found the roller massage group displayed significantly reduced soreness and greater pressure pain threshold compared with the control group at 0, 10 and 30 minutes post-massage.

Furthermore, positive results were found in a double-blind, randomised, controlled study by Romero-Moraleda et al. (2017), involving 32 participants. Both treatments (neurodynamic mobilisation and foam rolling) proved to be effective in reducing pain perception after DOMS, whereas only foam rolling application showed differences for the MVIC in the rectus femoris and isometric leg strength ($p < 0.01$). This was also the case when the effects of 20 minutes of foam rolling immediately, 24, and 48 hours post-exercise on the pressure-pain threshold, sprint speed (30 m sprint time), power (broad-jump distance), change-of-direction speed (T-test) and dynamic strength-endurance were analysed by Pearcey et al. (2015). Foam rolling effectively reduced DOMS and associated decrements in most dynamic performance measures. And finally, following high-intensity interval training (HIIT), the results from a study by Laffaye et al. (2019) indicated foam rolling did not impact the recovery of biomechanical variables, but did decrease DOMS and increased active and passive range of motion for the hip after HIIT, leading the authors to conclude that practitioners could use foam rolling to decrease muscle soreness after HIIT.

Is Pressure When Rolling Important?

Foam rolling cannot produce the same effects as those seen in myofascial release due to the method of application, as it is unlikely that enough force can be applied for the necessary physiological mechanisms to occur. In addition, in myofascial release the feedback from the therapist's hands and the pressure applied to the area being treated is more important than the amount of force applied. In one study on the forces required to elicit mechanical changes in fascia, Threlkeld (1992) noted some, but not all, permanent elongation in fascia begins when it is deformed to 3% of its initial length, and the mass component of force required to produce this change was between 24–115 kg. Therefore, actual tissue deformation would be painful and unachievable by foam rolling alone. Chaudhry et al. (2008) indicated that deformation forces which occur during manual therapy (in Newtons per mm^2) are not sufficient to cause a permanent change in solid connective tissue, such as the lumbar fascia, plantar fascia or the iliotibial ligament. Therefore, the palpable sensations of tissue release that are often reported by osteopathic physicians and other manual therapists cannot be due to deformations produced in the tissues. Sullivan et al. (2013) found that when the hamstrings were rolled, the average mass component of force exerted by using the opposing leg was only 13 kg. Greater amounts of pressure are rarely used when athletes foam roll. Curran et al. (2008) attempted to calculate the pressure exerted on soft tissue by two different types of foam rollers. It was determined that foam rollers made of harder material were significantly better in increasing soft tissue pressure and isolating the contact area. This study took its measurements in kilopascals and did not provide enough information for the values to be converted into kilograms, so it cannot be compared to the results of Threlkeld's (1992) and Sullivan et al.'s (2013) studies. By contrast, Murray et al. (2016) found the average foam rolling force of 68% of each subject's body weight increased the combination of hip and quadricep flexibility ($p = 0.03$; 2.4 degrees) following 60 seconds of foam rolling. Interestingly, muscle contractility was affected ($p = 0.09$–0.93), but temperature was not increased by foam rolling across time points ($p = 0.19$).

In summary, the wide range in study protocols with different measured outcomes relating to the type of roller used, the amount of pressure that needs to be applied and the length of time the limb should be rolled make results difficult to interpret. However, at this stage it does appear that pre-exercise foam rolling increases range of motion, through increased temperature changes and altered reflex sensitivity. As a recovery tool, post-exercise studies have been mostly positive on delayed onset muscle soreness symptom relief, possibly due to increased blood supply to connective tissue, but further studies are needed to confirm this.

Foam rolling techniques over the iliotibial band area are shown in Figure 11.2 and over the gastrocnemius in Figure 11.3.

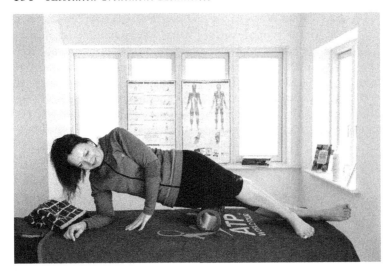

Figure 11.2 Iliotibial band.

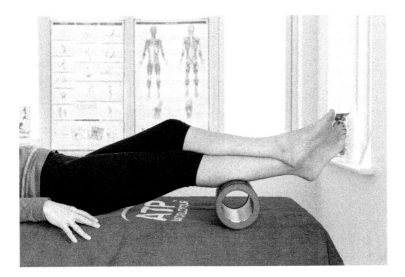

Figure 11.3 Gastrocnemius.

Instrument-Assisted Soft Tissue Massage/Fascial Abrasion Technique (Graston Technique®)

Graston Technique is a form of stainless steel instrument-assisted massage (IASTM) or fascial abrasion technique designed to release scar tissue, adhesions and fascial restrictions; it is shown in Figure 11.4. However, the research on its effectiveness has demonstrated mixed results, as the discussion in this section will outline. The instruments have either a convex or a concave shape. The concave shape allows for the pressure to be dispersed over a larger area, with the convex instrument applying pressure over a smaller surface area allowing the therapist to focus on more specific areas.

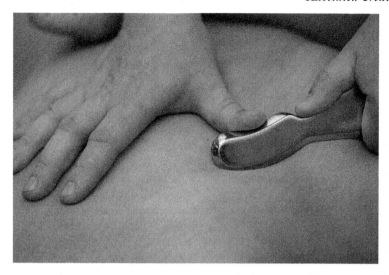

Figure 11.4 The instrument sweeps across the superficial fascia.

Research into instrument assisted massage has demonstrated positive effects on poste-rior shoulder range of motion (Laudner et al., 2014), dorsiflexion range of motion (Ikeda et al., 2019), chronic ankle instability and chronic calf pain (Bayliss et al., 2011), lumbar compartment syndrome (Hammer & Pfefer, 2005), tissue extensibility dysfunction (Baker et al., 2013) and Dupuytren's contracture (Christie et al., 2012). However, neutral effects to IASTM treatments have also been noted, including investigations into its effects on the properties of the plantar flexors (musculotendinous stiffness, passive range of motion, passive restive torque, maximal voluntary peak-torque) and on myofascial trigger points (Vardiman et al., 2015).

The Graston method of instrument-assisted soft tissue massage was compared to stick rolling massage in 16 college-aged males by Lee and colleagues (2020). The authors investigated the acute and residual effects of the two modalities on active and passive hamstring range of motion. The findings from this study demonstrated that both interventions were equally ben-eficial both immediately and over time. Basu et al. (2020) compared the effects of instrument-assisted soft tissue mobilisation and ischemic compression in upper trapezius trigger points in 30 badminton players. Each intervention was administered for a period of 2 weeks with two sessions per week in respective groups. Pre- and post-treatment assessments were taken measuring numeric pain rating scales (NPRS), pain pressure threshold and cervical range of motion. The authors' results indicated that there was a significant increase in the pain pressure threshold and cervical range of motion in the IASTM group. Additionally, there was a decrease in the NPRS findings in the IASTM group, suggesting that IASTM showed better results than ischemic compression in relieving trapezius trigger points.

Instrument-assisted soft tissue mobilisation (fascial abrasion) has been compared to foam rolling in the scientific community. Twenty soccer players had 2 minutes of rolling or instru-ment-assisted abrasions (IAB) to the quadriceps and hamstrings. Both groups significantly increased their range of motion (more so in the IAB group), but interestingly only the IAB group preserved most of these gains (7–13%) 24 hours later (Markovic, 2015). One study (Portillo-Soto et al., 2014) compared skin temperatures following 10 minutes of instrument-assisted soft tissue mobilisation or massage therapy in 28 participants. Both interventions increased skin temperature, which peaked at 25 minutes post-intervention. The authors believed this theoretically indicated an increase in blood flow.

Stroiney et al.'s (2020) study examined whether pre-exercise self-myofascial release and instrument-assisted soft tissue mobilisation would improve performance on measures of vertical jump height, 40-yard sprint time. Differences in perceived pain levels were also examined. In this particular study, the authors concluded that there was no interaction ($p > 0.05$) between the massage interventions and the sex of the participants for both the vertical jump and 40-yard sprint tests, and no significant difference in perceived pain (t [49] = -1.60, $p >$ 0.05). In another study analysing the effects of 3 minutes of IASTM treatment, in a protocol designed by MacDonald et al. (2016) measuring vertical jump height, peak power and peak velocity, no significant differences between treatment groups were found when using the current IASTM treatment parameters. The authors also highlighted the fact that drawing accurate conclusions on this topic is difficult, and more research is needed to determine the effect of IASTM on muscular performance. Gulick (2018) used a 5-minute intervention including three IASTM techniques to effectively increase the pressure pain threshold of a myofascial trigger point (MTrP) in the upper trapezius during six treatments over a 3-week period ($p <$ 0.0001). The outcomes from Lambert et al.'s (2017) systematic review (7 studies) supports the idea that IASTM may have an impact on physiological changes by providing an increase in blood flow, reduction in tissue viscosity, myofascial release, interruption of pain receptors and improvement of flexibility of underlying tissue. Therefore, the authors suggested that IASTM is an effective treatment intervention for reducing pain and improving function in less than a three-month period.

Furthermore, thirteen articles met the inclusion criteria in Seffrin et al.'s (2019) systematic review on instrument assisted soft tissue mobilisations. The authors stated that the current literature provides support for IASTM in improving ROM in uninjured individuals, as well as pain and patient-reported function (or both) in injured patients. More high-quality research involving a larger variety of patients and products is needed to further substantiate and allow for generalisation of these findings. However, as Kim et al. (2017) summarised, published articles consisting mostly of case reports rather than experimental studies, with some of the case reports failing to present the details of the IASTM protocol that was applied, make results difficult to interpret.

Dry Needling

Although not part of the sports massage syllabus, many therapists add dry needling to their skillset as it has a strong crossover with their manual therapy trigger point work. Dry needling utilises a thin solid filament needle to stimulate neuromuscular tissue to elicit a pain-reducing response versus a direct anti-inflammatory or muscular response mediated by the introduction of a drug into the trigger point (Boyce et al., 2020). It is shown in Figure 11.5.

The needle tip touches, taps or pricks tiny nerve endings or neural tissue (i.e. 'sensitive loci' or 'nociceptors') when it is inserted into a myofascial trigger point (Dunning et al., 2014), which may lead to a 'local twitch response' (LTR). The LTR is an involuntary spinal reflex contraction of muscle fibres within a taut band and occurs during needling. This LTR elicited by dry needling is associated with pain relief and a palpable reduction of muscle stiffness. It is visible and palpable and thought to occur in response to altered sensory spinal processing resulting from sensitised peripheral mechanical nociceptors by interrupting motor end plate noise, eliciting an analgesic effect (Hsieh et al., 2007). However, Perreault et al. (2017) concluded that the local twitch response appears unnecessary for managing myofascial pain and is unrelated to many of the positive effects of dry needling.

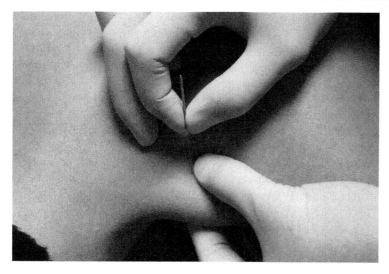

Figure 11.5 Closeup of dry needling technique in the upper trapezius.

In the last few years there has been a large number of systematic reviews and meta-analyses on the effects of dry needling, with the majority investigating its effects on myofascial trigger points and pain relief. Its effects in the upper trapezius area have been investigated (Ong & Claydon, 2014; Ziaeifar et al., 2014; Cagnie et al., 2015; Gerber et al., 2015; Liu et al., 2015; Hall et al., 2018), alongside studies of its use in treating head and neck pain (France et al., 2014; Sterling et al., 2015; Cerezo-Téllez et al., 2016; Kamali et al., 2019), lower back pain (Hu et al., 2018), jaw pain (Fernández-Carnero et al., 2010; Vier et al., 2019) and in other less specific areas, including the lower quarter (Morihisa et al., 2016), multiple body regions (Boyles et al., 2015), musculoskeletal conditions (Gattie et al., 2017), pain and disability (Jackson et al., 2016) and in the effectiveness of blinding in the moderation of pain outcomes (Braithwaite et al., 2018).

Positive short-term outcomes have been found by Liu et al. (2015), although wet needling was found to be more effective than dry needling for relieving pain from MTrPs in the neck and shoulders in the medium term. Morihisa et al., (2016) suggested dry needling was effective in reducing pain associated with lower quarter trigger points in the short term. However, their findings suggested dry needling does not have a positive effect on function, quality of life, depression, range of motion or strength. Cagnie et al. (2015) concluded both dry needling and ischemic compression could be recommended for treating trigger points. In another study, again highlighting positive outcomes, Gerber et al. (2015) found dry needling reduces pain and changes myofascial trigger point status. In addition, improvements in pain intensity, pressure pain threshold and disability of arm, hand and shoulder (DASH) were found and may be prescribed for subjects with trigger points in upper trapezius muscles. especially when pain relief is the goal of the treatment (Ziaeifar et al., 2014).

Further research has indicated positive results, with Cerezo-Telez et al. (2016) noting deep dry needling and passive stretching are more effective than passive stretching alone in people with non-specific neck pain. Boyles et al.'s (2015) review showed a measured benefit from trigger point dry needling for MTrPs in multiple body areas, suggesting broad applicability of trigger point dry needling treatment for multiple muscle groups. A review of the literature by Vier et al. (2019) demonstrated dry needling is better than other interventions for pain intensity as well as being more effective than sham therapy on pressure pain threshold. However, the authors concluded that there is very low-quality evidence and a small effect size. The quality of research was also highlighted by Gattie et al. (2017), who suggested there was very low-quality to moderate-quality evidence that in the immediate to 12-week follow-up period dry needling is more effective than no treatment, sham dry needling and other treatments for reducing pain and improving pressure pain threshold in patients presenting with musculoskeletal pain. The authors concluded that no differences in functional outcomes exist when compared to other physical therapy treatments. Sterling et al. (2015), who found no effects from dry needling (or exercise) on subjects with whiplash injuries, concurred. Therefore, although the results on the effectiveness of dry needling seem to be mostly positive, as with any other treatment modality it may improve symptoms for some, but not all.

Cupping

In addition to treatment goals of decreasing musculoskeletal pain, cupping therapy in sports medicine, sometimes referred to as myofascial decompression, is utilised to increase range of motion by using glass or plastic cups along with fire or a vacuum pump to create a negative pressure on the applied body regions (Schafer et al., 2020). The technique is shown in Figure 11.6.

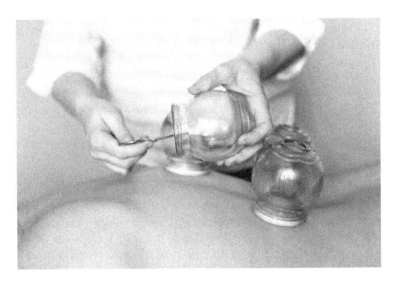

Figure 11.6 Fire cupping cups on the back of a patient.

Results from eleven trials with 498 participants from China, the United States, Greece, Iran, and the United Arab Emirates were included in a systematic review by Bridgett et al. (2018). The authors reported the effects on different populations, including footballers, handball players, swimmers, gymnasts and track and field athletes, of both amateur and professional nature. Cupping was applied between one and 20 times, in daily or weekly intervals, alone or in combination with, for example, acupuncture. The authors concluded that cupping was beneficial for perceptions of pain and disability, increased range of motion and reductions in creatine kinase (CK) when compared to mostly untreated control groups, but the majority of the studies had an unclear or high risk of bias. In an earlier systematic review addressing the effects of cupping for treating pain, Kim et al. (2009) suggested there was evidence for the effectiveness of cupping in the management of pain conditions. However, the total number of randomised controlled trials ($n = 7$) included in their analysis and the methodological quality were too low to draw firm conclusions.

Lederer et al. (2019) measured tissue stiffness in 40 participants with chronic back and neck pain using a myometer. The results from this study suggested that pain relief after cupping massage cannot be explained by reducing tissue stiffness (as this returned to baseline in 24 hours, and pain was as before), which led the authors to make a valuable point that the intensity of pain might not be related to increased stiffness of the myometrically measurable myofascial tissue. Pain improvement by cupping seems to be induced on a more systemic level. In 25 healthy individuals, 10 minutes of cupping (compared to sham cupping and control) did not improve hamstring flexibility in a study by Schafer et al. (2020). These results were in agreement with those of Williams et al. (2019), who confirmed that cupping demonstrated no statistically significant changes in hamstring flexibility in 25 college soccer players.

In a study by Volpato et al. (2020), patients with back pain showed a significant improvement in all pain severity items and sleep in the brief pain inventory ($p < 0.05$) and a decrease in disability in the Rolande Morris disability questionnaire ($p < 0.001$). No significant differences were found in pressure pain threshold or skin temperature. Thus, the authors concluded, cupping therapy is effective in reducing low back pain and decreasing disability after one single session but not in changing skin mechanical threshold or temperature. In addition, 16 studies were included in the qualitative analysis and ten in the quantitative analysis in Moura et al.'s (2018) systematic review and meta-analysis. Cupping therapy demonstrated positive results on chronic back pain. The authors noted there is no standardisation in the treatment protocols. The main assessed outcomes were pain intensity, physical incapacity, quality of life and nociceptive threshold before the mechanical stimulus. There was a significant reduction in the pain intensity score through the use of cupping therapy ($p = 0.001$). Therefore, it can be concluded that while cupping therapy may provide relief for those with (back) pain, it is unlikely to provide increases in range of motion

Cryotherapy

Using cold as a means of physical treatment is a practice that has been studied and utilised since the age of the ancient Egyptians 4,000 years ago. They noted that the application of cold was effective in minimising the pain of trauma and decreasing inflammation (Saini, 2015).

Cryotherapy (Figure 11.7) is frequently used by athletes as a post-exercise recovery intervention to relieve pain, reduce muscle spasm and minimise inflammation following strenuous exercise. The mechanism of cold therapy for recovery after exercise is predominantly attributed to its deep state of vasoconstrictive effect (Khoshnevis et al., 2015) which reduces inflammation reaction through a decrease of the cell metabolism. There are a number of methods of applying cryotherapy; these include cold water immersion (CWI) (ice baths), cold chambers (cold air exposure), cryo-cuffs, crushed ice (wrapped in a towel or a bag) and ice or gel packs.

Becoming increasingly popular, cold water immersion is one of the most common methods of cryotherapy and is used to minimise fatigue, induce vasoconstriction, stimulate venous return, aid metabolite removal after exercise and reduce swelling and muscle soreness for faster recovery. Another method used is whole body cryotherapy (WBC): this involves exposing individuals to extremely cold dry air, which means below −100°C, for two to four minutes in a specialised cabin or chamber. It is thought to work through reductions in muscle, skin and core temperature which stimulate cutaneous receptors

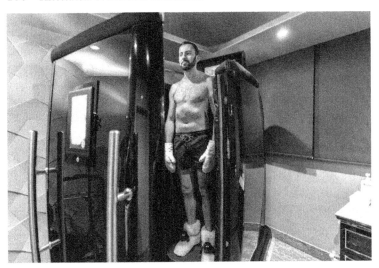

Figure 11.7 Man taking cryotherapy treatment, standing at the capsule door.

and excite the sympathetic adrenergic fibres, causing constriction of local blood vessels (Costello et al., 2014).

A study by Ishan et al. (2016) indicated that CWI application appears to demonstrate limited recovery benefits when exercise-induced muscle damage was induced by single-joint eccentrically biased contractions. However, it appears to be more effective in ameliorating the effects of EIMD induced by whole-body prolonged endurance/intermittent based exercise modalities. Peake and colleagues (2017) found cold water immersion is no more effective than an active recovery for reducing inflammation or cellular stress in muscle following a bout of resistance exercise. These findings were corroborated by de Freitas et al. (2019), who demonstrated that the results of 5 continuous days of CWI (after training) indicated limited effects on performance, muscle damage, inflammation markers and reactive oxygen species mediators in 12 volleyball players. In addition, Grainger et al. (2020) found that partial body cryotherapy did not improve restoration of selected performance parameters (sleep, DOMS, countermovement jump) in 18 professional rugby union players. Furthermore, a study using recreational street runners (Dantas et al., 2020), showed that ten minutes of CWI at 10°C was no more effective than water immersion or rest in recovering triple hop distance and peak extension torque. Leeder et al. (2019) found that CWI provides limited benefits in attenuating the deleterious effects experienced during tournament scenarios, but the treatment was associated with faster sprint times 24 hours after the tournament scenario. By contrast, in 28 professional basket players who received cold water immersion following training and matches over a season, all serum muscular markers (except myoglobin) were higher in the cold water immersion group than the control group ($p < 0.05$). The time course of changes in muscle markers over the season also differed between the groups ($p < 0.05$). In the cold water immersion group, ratings of perceived exertion decreased significantly. Isokinetic torque differed between the groups at the end of the season (60 o/s peak torque: $p < 0.001$ and $\eta^2 p$: 0.884; and 180 o/s peak torque: $p < 0.001$ and $\eta^2 p$: 0.898) had changed significantly over the season in the cold water immersion group ($p < 0.05$) (Seco-Calvo et al., 2020). Nine studies were included for a review and meta-analysis by Machado et al. (2016). The authors noted the available evidence suggests CWI can be slightly better than passive recovery in the management of muscle soreness. Their results also demonstrated the presence of a dose-response relationship, indicating that CWI with a water temperature of between 11 and 15°C and an immersion time of 11–15 minutes can provide the best results.

Comparing different cryotherapy recovery methods in a small sample (eight elite junior cyclists), Chan et al. (2016) investigated the effects of cold water immersion, cold compression therapy (CCT) and 15 minutes of active recovery (ACT). The authors highlighted no significant difference between average power output, blood lactate, rating of perceived exertion and heart rate in two time-trial bouts for all recovery interventions. Therefore, they could all be used as recovery methods between exercise bouts and could be selected by availability and personal preference. Additionally, 13 studies were examined in a systematic review on the effects of cryotherapy methods on circulatory, metabolic, inflammatory and neural properties (Freire et al., 2016). The authors concluded that cryotherapy promotes a significant decrease in blood flow, venous capillary pressure, oxygen saturation and haemoglobin (only for superficial tissues) and nerve conduction velocity. However, the effect of cryotherapy on the concentration of inflammatory substances induced by exercise (creatine kinase enzyme and myoglobin) remains unclear.

Depth of water during cold water immersion has been thought to play an important role due to the increased hydrostatic pressure on the musculature in deeper water. Interestingly, with every 1 metre of immersion, the pressure gradient rises by 74 mm Hg (mm Hg = millimetres of mercury) – almost equal to typical diastolic blood pressure (80 mm Hg) (Wilcock et al., 2006). Leeder et al. (2015) compared seated and standing CWI and discovered that seated cold water immersion was associated with lower DOMS than standing cold water immersion (effect size = 1.86; $p = 0.001$).

Using a small sample ($n = 10$), Abaïdia et al. (2017) investigated recovery from exercise-induced muscle damage via cold water immersion compared to whole-body cryotherapy. Although only small effects were found, CWI was more effective than WBC in accelerating recovery kinetics for countermovement-jump performance at 72 hours post-exercise. Cold water immersion also demonstrated lower soreness and higher perceived recovery levels 24–48 hours post-exercise. Although the muscle-damaging protocols were different, Hohenauer et al. (2018) found cold water immersion had a greater impact on the physiological response (thigh muscle oxygen saturation, mean arterial pressure, local skin temperature, cutaneous vascular conductance) than to partial body cryotherapy. The 36 articles in Hohenauer et al.'s earlier systematic review and meta-analysis (2015) on the effect of post-exercise cryotherapy on recovery characteristics (DOMS up to 96 hrs and rate of perceived exertion [RPE] up to 24 hrs) revealed that cooling is superior compared to passive recovery strategies after various exhaustive or muscle-damaging exercise protocols. The length of time of cold water submersion, the depth of water and the body fat of the individual vary greatly within the literature; however, in Hohenauer et al.'s (2015) review, the mean temperature showed a significant result favouring cooling at 10°C (range: 5°C to 13°C) compared to the passive recovery intervention. The authors suggested the cooling time for alleviating the subjective symptoms was 13 minutes (range: 10 minutes to 24 minutes).

In Costello and colleagues' (2016) Cochrane review of 4 studies on whole-body cryotherapy (extreme cold air exposure) for preventing and treating muscle soreness after exercise, the authors concluded that whole-body cryotherapy does not effectively reduce muscle soreness or improve subjective recovery after exercise in physically active young men. In agreement, Wilson et al. (2019) suggested that WBC is more effective than cold water immersion, but neither was more effective than a placebo in accelerating recovery. In comparison, study designs within the articles retrieved in Rose et al.'s (2017) review of the literature on whole-body cryotherapy as a recovery technique after exercise were vastly different, making inferences across studies difficult. However, the authors concluded from their review that WBC may be successful in enhancing maximal voluntary contractions and returning athletes to pre-exercise strength at a faster rate. With WBC treatment conditions recording pain scores on average 31% lower than control groups, the evidence tends to favour WBC as an analgesic treatment after damaging exercise, indicated by a potential dampening of the inflammatory cytokine response. This concurs with Qu and colleagues (2020). The authors compared cold water immersion, contrast-water therapy (CWT) and whole-body cryotherapy, and found that WBC positively affected muscle soreness and muscle recovery and affected the visual analogue score (VAS), creatine kinase, C-reactive protein (CRP) activity and vertical jump height (VJH) associated with exercised induced muscle damage. Therefore, for middle- and long-distance runners with EIMD, WBC exerts better recovery effects than CWI, CWT and the control group (CON) immediately post-exercise, and at 1, 24, 48, 72 and 96 hours later.

Twenty elite wrestlers participated in a study (Demirhan et al., 2015) investigating the effects of 8 minutes of ice massage vs cold water immersion on delayed onset muscle soreness and creatine kinase levels. The results of this revealed that significant differences were observed within both groups at all times ($p < 0.001$) (DOMS at 24 and 48 hours). Adamczyk et al. (2016) also investigated ice massage and cold water immersion ($n = 36$) and concluded both modalities showed positive results in utilising lactate and preventing DOMS, thereby supporting post-exercise recovery. The novel approach of examining the effects of combining myofascial release with ice application on a latent trigger point in the forearm in young adults was performed by Gutiérrez-Rojas et al. (2015). Echoing the results of Adamczyk et al. (2016) and those of Demirhan et al. (2015), the authors concluded that there were immediate improvements in pain variables after the application of ice massage. However, Howatson et al. (2005) applied 15 minutes of ice cup massage to the elbow flexors in 12 physically active males following eccentric exercise to induce delayed onset muscle soreness. The authors found ice massage to be ineffective in reducing the indirect markers of DOMS and did not improve recovery in muscle function. In contrast, Anaya-Terroba et al. (2010) noted ice massage after isokinetic exercise produced an immediate increase to the pressure pain threshold of the vastus lateralis (VL), vastus medialis (VM) and EMG activity, suggesting that ice massage has a hypoallergenic effect and improves EMG activity. A study involving 11 college-aged male volunteers using isometric contractions performed every 2 minutes for 20 minutes yielded neutral results on muscle force output following 10 minutes of ice massage applied over the right bicep muscle belly (Borgmeyer et al., 2004).

And finally, the findings from a study using 16 recreationally trained men (DuPont et al., 2017) undergoing a combination of cold and compression therapy for 20 minutes immediately after exercise and then 24 and 48 hours later indicated that it was an effective method to help recovery from an acute bout of intense resistance exercise. It is possible, as the results of this study indicated, that less muscle damage occurred as measured indirectly using serum creatine kinase concentrations, but the perceptual feeling of recovery and soreness cannot be ignored.

It would appear that CWI demonstrates mixed results largely due to the inconsistencies in depth of water, time submerged, temperature selected and body fat of the individual. Whole body cryotherapy has also yielded mixed results, although it does appear it may be beneficial in reducing inflammatory markers from exercise-induced muscle damage. Ice massage has also demonstrated equivocal findings however it may provide some pain relief, at least in the short term.

During exposure to cold therapy treatments, some athletes experience adverse effects to the modality. This may include constant shivering, confusion, irregular pulse rate, a decrease in blood pressure, fatigue and loss of circulation. It is also important to take precautions regarding skin burns when using ice or gel packs. A barrier (wet towel or wrap) should be used, rather than applying ice directly onto the skin.

Contraindications to Cryotherapy

- Poor circulation (cardiac conditions, Raynaud's).
- Open wounds or damaged skin.
- Where there is limited circulation (diabetes, nerve injuries causing reduced or loss of sensation).
- Urticaria (hives due to extreme cold exposure).

Contrast Water Therapy

Contrast water therapy (CWT) is frequently used by the athletic population as another means of recovery from strenuous exercise. It has been speculated that CWT reduces oedema through a 'pumping action' that is created by vasoconstriction and vasodilation and reduces muscle spasm, pain and inflammation, and increases range of motion. However, there is a lack of scientific evidence to support its effectiveness and the correct protocol to be used.

Bieuzen and colleagues' (2013) systematic review and meta-analysis examined the literature (18 studies) on the effects of contrast water therapy on exercise-induced muscle damage. The authors concluded, despite the high risk of bias, that data from 13 studies showed that CWT resulted in significantly greater improvements in muscle soreness at the five follow-up time points (< 6, 24, 48, 72 and 96 hours) in comparison to passive recovery. Pooled data also showed CWT significantly reduced muscle strength loss at each follow-up time (< 6, 24, 48, 72 and 96 hours) in comparison to passive recovery. In an earlier study on the effects of CWT, positive results were also found by Vaile et al. (2007) when contrast water therapy was compared to passive recovery. The authors' results indicated smaller reduction and faster restoration of strength and power, measured by isometric force and jump squat production following DOMS-inducing leg-press exercise, when compared to passive recovery. Twenty-three peer reviewed articles ($n = 606$) were included in Higgins et al.'s (2017) systematic review and meta-analysis examining the effects of cold water immersion and contrast water therapy for recovery from team sports. The results indicated CWI was beneficial for recovery (countermovement jump, $p = 0.05$, CI –0.004–0.578; all-out sprint, $p = 0.02$, CI –0.056–0.801). The cold water immersion also proved to be beneficial for recovery at 72 hours (fatigue: $p = 0.03$, CI 0.061–1.418) and contrast water therapy was beneficial for recovery at 48 hours (fatigue: $p = 0.04$, CI 0.013–0.942).

A contrast water therapy group consisting of periodic immersions in cold water (18°C) for 1 minute and then in hot water (37°C) for 2 minutes, with accumulating 15 minutes in the water compared to a recovery of slow jogging (SJR) for 8 minutes (6.8 km · h^{-1}) (Pelana et al., 2019). Results indicated after a 30-minute recovery, lactate concentration was significantly greater ($p = 0.001$) in the SJR group (7.67 mmol/l) than in the CWT group (6.82 mmol/l) and remained significantly different 60 minutes after recovery ($p = 0.0001$; 6.80 mmol/l and 5.01 mmol/l, respectively). Therefore, in elite futsal players, CWT had an effect on recovery by decreasing lactate concentration and rapid recovery of heart rate.

Compression Garments

Compression garments (CG) on the lower limbs are increasingly popular among athletes who wish to improve performance, reduce exercise-induced discomfort and reduce the risk of injury

(Beliard et al., 2015). However, results from scientific studies on the effectiveness of using upper and lower body compression garments and devices to recover from strenuous exercise is difficult to interpret, due to the varying training status of the participants, when they are used, the type of exercise performed before use, the design of the compression garments tested and the amount and duration of pressure applied.

Twenty-three peer-reviewed studies, using healthy participants, were reviewed in Brown et al.'s (2017) meta-analysis examining the use of compression garments and recovery from exercise. The results from this study indicated strength recovery was subject to greater benefits than other outcomes ($p < 0.001$), displaying large, very likely benefits at 2–8 hours ($p < 0.001$) and > 24 hours ($p < 0.001$). Investigating the effects of compression garments for the recovery of exercise-induced muscle damage, Marques-Jimenez et al.'s (2016) systematic review and meta-analysis revealed that despite controversy in pressure, time of treatment and type of garments, there was evidence CG reduced perceived muscle soreness and swelling, increased power and strength. However, the treatment had no effect in decreasing lactate or creatine kinase, and provided little evidence of decreasing lactate dehydrogenase. Therefore, the authors suggested that the application of compression clothing may aid in the recovery of exercise-induced muscle damage. In another study by the same author, Marques-Jimenez et al. (2018) concluded wearing compression garments can be useful between 24–48 hours post-exercise to promote psychological recovery and could also have a positive effect on aerobic capacity, although the placebo effect could not be ruled out. In another positive article (Broatch et al., 2018) investigating cycling performance ($n = 20$) revealed compression garments improved muscle blood flow (vastus lateralis) and exercise performance during repeated-sprint cycling. Furthermore, Beliard et al. (2015) reviewed the literature (24 articles were selected) to determine the beneficial effects of compression and to evaluate whether there is any relationship between the pressure applied and the reported effects. From their review, the researchers concluded wearing compression garments during recovery from exercise seems to be beneficial for performance recovery and DOMS, but the factors affecting this efficacy remain to be elucidated; the value and spatial pattern of the pressure applied had no influence on the results.

Other findings were not so positive, including a study of 55 articles involving 788 participants which was discussed in a review by Engel et al. (2016). The authors concluded compression clothing has no significant impact on performance parameters during running, ice speed skating, triathlon, cross country skiing and kayaking. However, wearing compression clothing might improve cycling performance, reduce post-exercise muscle pain following running and cycling and facilitate lactate elimination during recovery. This was corroborated by Govus et al. (2018), who found neither compression garments nor neuromuscular electrical stimulation promoted physiological or perceptual recovery following sprint competition in cross country skiers, compared with a control group.

To summarise, it appears compression garments could be a valuable tool in athletic recovery by reducing some of the negative effects caused by exercise-induced muscle damage, although as previously mentioned, due to the varying training status of the participants, the type of exercise performed, the design of the compression garments tested and the amount of pressure applied, results are difficult to interpret. However, it should be noted that the positive effects of compression garments on perceptual soreness and feeling of recovery should not be overlooked (placebo).

Heat Treatments/Thermotherapy

Heat can be applied either pre- or post-performance, or as a treatment modality, by using hot packs, sauna, warm/hot water submersion (hot bath) or topical lotions. Heat therapy has demonstrated therapeutic benefits for both analgesia and reducing muscle tonicity (Nadler et al., 2004); it causes vasodilation in the veins, facilitating the removal of lactate from muscle tissue to be converted back into pyruvic acid in the liver with the help of lactate dehydrogenase (Putra et al., 2020). Thermotherapy can be used as monotherapy or in combination with oral analgesics to relieve acute low back pain and muscle soreness (Nadler et al., 2002) and, when combined with a combination of multi-disciplinary treatment, may be a promising method for the treatment of chronic pain (Masuda et al., 2005). Similarly, positive results were found by Mayer et al. (2005). The authors stated that by combining continuous low-level heat wrap therapy with directional preference-based exercise during the treatment of acute low back pain, significant improvements in functional outcomes were found compared with either intervention alone or control. Furthermore, a programme of thermotherapy using hot packs for 20 minutes (in prone lying position) was compared to posterior-anterior vertebral mobilisations (PAVMs) in a study on non-specific back pain (NSLBP) (Baig et al., 2018). The authors concluded both have significant effects on NSLBP in terms of relieving pain and improving functional disability. However, PAVMs appeared to be more effective than thermotherapy.

Petrofsky et al. (2017) discovered heat works well when applied immediately after DOMS-inducing exercise, but not 24 hours later, demonstrating that once there is cellular disruption in muscle, damage has occurred and is hard to stop. This indicates that much less muscle damage occurs when heat is applied immediately after exercise. In agreement, Kim et al.'s, (2019) results showed exposure to heat therapy (5 × daily for 90 minutes) immediately and for 4 consecutive days after a maximal bout of eccentric exercise hastens recovery of fatigue resistance, reduces perceived soreness and promotes the expression of angiogenic factors in human skeletal muscle.

In a study by Cernych et al. (2019), post-sauna recovery was accompanied by slowed salivary free cortisol diurnal kinetics, whereas noradrenaline, dopamine and serotonin did not persist into the second hour of recovery after the sauna. Although recovery to normothermia after a sauna led to a greater acceleration of muscle contractility properties and decreased muscle steadiness, sustained isometric submaximal contraction did not provoke greater neuromuscular fatigability. Negative results were noted in swimmers who performed significantly worse after a sauna (SAU) (4 × 50-metre pre–post difference: +1.69 seconds) than after placebo (PLAC) (–0.66 seconds; $p = 0.02$), with the most pronounced decrease in the first 50 metre ($p = 0.04$; +2.7 seconds). Overall performance of 15 athletes deteriorated (+2.6 seconds). The subjective feeling of stress was significantly higher after SAU than after PLAC ($p = 0.03$). Therefore, at least in competitive swimmers, sauna does not appear to be a valuable asset for sports performance (Skorski et al., 2019). In addition, following sub-maximal exercise, Putra et al. (2020) concluded that the reduction in blood lactic acid levels with warm water recovery (temperature 35°C–37°C) proved to be greater than in their aromatherapy sauna recovery group.

Contraindications to Heat Treatment/Thermotherapy

- Recent haemorrhage.
- Skin infection.
- Recent fever or infection.
- Vascular disease (DVT, diabetic complications).
- Confused or unreliable patients.

With some conditions, such as pregnancy, acute inflammation and superficial metal implants, heat should not be used, or used only with a physician's approval. Of note, one study by

Batavia (2004) found no reports of metal implant-related complications in the literature, so heat could be applied with caution to local areas. However, from the above studies, heat (excluding sauna) appears to be a useful modality in hastening recovery from delayed onset muscle soreness and low back pain or discomfort, and therefore its use should be considered by athletes and therapists.

References

Abaïdia, A.E., Lamblin, J., Delecroix, B., Leduc, C., McCall, A., Nédélec, M., Dawson, B., Baquet, G. and Dupont, G., 2017. Recovery from exercise-induced muscle damage: Cold-water immersion versus whole-body cryotherapy. *International Journal of Sports Physiology and Performance*, 12(3), pp. 402–409.

Adamczyk, J.G., Krasowska, I., Boguszewski, D. and Reaburn, P., 2016. The use of thermal imaging to assess the effectiveness of ice massage and cold-water immersion as methods for supporting post-exercise recovery. *Journal of Thermal Biology*, 60, pp. 20–25.

Anaya-Terroba, L., Arroyo-Morales, M., Fernández-de-las-Peñas, C., Díaz-Rodríguez, L. and Cleland, J.A., 2010. Effects of ice massage on pressure pain thresholds and electromyography activity postexercise: A randomized controlled crossover study. *Journal of Manipulative and Physiological Therapeutics*, 33(3), pp. 212–219.

Baig, A.A.M., Ahmed, S.I., Ali, S.S., Rahmani, A. and Siddiqui, F., 2018. Role of posterior-anterior vertebral mobilization versus thermotherapy in non-specific lower back pain. *Pakistan Journal of Medical Sciences*, 34(2), p. 435.

Baker, R.T., Nasypany, A., Seegmiller, J.G. and Baker, J.G., 2013. Instrument-assisted soft tissue mobilization treatment for tissue extensibility dysfunction. *International Journal of Athletic Therapy and Training*, 18(5), pp. 16–21.

Basu, S., Edgaonkar, R., Baxi, G., Palekar, T.J., Vijayakumar, M., Swami, A. and Tai, M.Z., 2020. Comparative study of instrument assisted soft tissue mobilisation vs ischemic compression in myofascial trigger points on upper trapezius muscle in professional badminton players. *Indian Journal of Physiotherapy & Occupational Therapy*, 14(1), pp. 253–258.

Batavia, M., 2004. Contraindications for superficial heat and therapeutic ultrasound: Do sources agree? *Archives of Physical Medicine and Rehabilitation*, 85(6), pp. 1006–1012.

Bayliss, A.J., Klene, F.J., Gundeck, E.L. and Loghmani, M.T., 2011. Treatment of a patient with post-natal chronic calf pain utilizing instrument-assisted soft tissue mobilization: A case study. *Journal of Manual & Manipulative Therapy*, 19(3), pp. 127–134.

Behara, B. and Jacobson, B.H., 2017. Acute effects of deep tissue foam rolling and dynamic stretching on muscular strength, power, and flexibility in division I linemen. *The Journal of Strength & Conditioning Research*, 31(4), pp. 888–892.

Behm, D.G. and Wilke, J., 2019. Do self-myofascial release devices release myofascia? Rolling mechanisms: A narrative review. *Sports Medicine*, 49(8), pp. 1173–1181.

Beliard, S., Chauveau, M., Moscatiello, T., Cros, F., Ecarnot, F. and Becker, F., 2015. Compression garments and exercise: No influence of pressure applied. *Journal of Sports Science & Medicine*, 14(1), p. 75.

Bieuzen, F., Bleakley, C.M. and Costello, J.T., 2013. Contrast water therapy and exercise induced muscle damage: A systematic review and meta-analysis. *PLoS One*, 8(4), p. e62356.

Borgmeyer, J.A., Scott, B.A. and Mayhew, J.L., 2004. The effects of ice massage on maximum isokinetic-torque production. *Journal of Sport Rehabilitation*, 13(1), pp. 1–8.

Boyce, D., Wempe, H., Campbell, C., Fuehne, S., Zylstra, E., Smith, G., Wingard, C. and Jones, R., 2020. Adverse events associated with therapeutic dry needling. *International Journal of Sports Physical Therapy*, 15(1), p. 103.

Boyles, R., Fowler, R., Ramsey, D. and Burrows, E., 2015. Effectiveness of trigger point dry needling for multiple body regions: A systematic review. *Journal of Manual & Manipulative Therapy*, 23(5), pp. 276–293.

Braithwaite, F.A., Walters, J.L., Li, L.S.K., Moseley, G.L., Williams, M.T. and McEvoy, M.P., 2018. Effectiveness and adequacy of blinding in the moderation of pain outcomes: Systematic review and meta-analyses of dry needling trials. *PeerJ, 6*, p. e5318.

Bridgett, R., Klose, P., Duffield, R., Mydock, S. and Lauche, R., 2018. Effects of cupping therapy in amateur and professional athletes: Systematic review of randomized controlled trials. *The Journal of Alternative and Complementary Medicine, 24*(3), pp. 208–219.

Broatch, J.R., Bishop, D.J. and Halson, S., 2018. Lower limb sports compression garments improve muscle blood flow and exercise performance during repeated-sprint cycling. *International Journal of Sports Physiology and Performance, 13*(7), pp. 882–890.

Brown, F., Gissane, C., Howatson, G., Van Someren, K., Pedlar, C. and Hill, J., 2017. Compression garments and recovery from exercise: A meta-analysis. *Sports Medicine, 47*(11), pp. 2245–2267.

Cagnie, B., Castelein, B., Pollie, F., Steelant, L., Verhoeyen, H. and Cools, A., 2015. Evidence for the use of ischemic compression and dry needling in the management of trigger points of the upper trapezius in patients with neck pain: A systematic review. *American Journal of Physical Medicine & Rehabilitation, 94*(7), pp. 573–583.

Cerezo-Téllez, E., Torres-Lacomba, M., Fuentes-Gallardo, I., Perez-Muñoz, M., Mayoral-del-Moral, O., Lluch-Girbés, E., Prieto-Valiente, L. and Falla, D., 2016. Effectiveness of dry needling for chronic nonspecific neck pain: A randomized, single-blinded, clinical trial. *Pain, 157*(9), pp. 1905–1917.

Cernych, M., Baranauskiene, N., Vitkauskiene, A., Satas, A. and Brazaitis, M., 2019. Accelerated muscle contractility and decreased muscle steadiness following sauna recovery do not induce greater neuromuscular fatigability during sustained submaximal contractions. *Human Movement Science, 63*, pp. 10–19.

Chan, Y.Y., Yim, Y.M., Bercades, D., Cheng, T.T., Ngo, K.L. and Lo, K.K., 2016. Comparison of different cryotherapy recovery methods in elite junior cyclists. *Asia-Pacific Journal of Sports Medicine, Arthroscopy, Rehabilitation and Technology, 5*, pp. 17–23.

Chaudhry, H., Bukiet, B. and Findley, T., 2008. Mathematical analysis of applied loads on skeletal muscles during manual therapy. *The Journal of the American Osteopathic Association, 108*(12), pp. 680–688.

Cheatham, S.W., Stull, K.R. and Kolber, M.J., 2019. Comparison of a vibration roller and a non-vibration roller intervention on knee range of motion and pressure pain threshold: A randomized controlled trial. *Journal of Sport Rehabilitation, 28*(1), pp. 39–45.

Christie, W.S., Puhl, A.A. and Lucaciu, O.C., 2012. Cross-frictional therapy and stretching for the treatment of palmar adhesions due to Dupuytren's contracture: A prospective case study. *Manual Therapy, 17*(5), pp. 479–482.

Costello, J., Donnelly, A., Karki, A. and Selfe, J., 2014. Effects of whole-body cryotherapy and cold-water immersion on knee skin temperature. *International Journal of Sports Medicine, 35*(1), pp. 35–40.

Costello, J.T., Baker, P.R., Minett, G.M., Bieuzen, F., Stewart, I.B. and Bleakley, C., 2016. Cochrane review: Whole-body cryotherapy (extreme cold air exposure) for preventing and treating muscle soreness after exercise in adults. *Journal of Evidence-Based Medicine, 9*(1), pp. 43–44.

Couture, G., Karlik, D., Glass, S.C. and Hatzel, B.M., 2015. The effect of foam rolling duration on hamstring range of motion. *The Open Orthopaedics Journal, 9*, p. 450.

Curran, P.F., Fiore, R.D. and Crisco, J.J., 2008. A comparison of the pressure exerted on soft tissue by 2 myofascial rollers. *Journal of Sport Rehabilitation, 17*(4), pp. 432–442.

D'Amico, A., Gillis, J., McCarthy, K., Leftin, J., Molloy, M., Heim, H. and Burke, C. 2020. Foam rolling and indices of autonomic recovery following exercise-induced muscle damage. *International Journal of Sports Physical Therapy, 15*(3), p. 429.

Dantas, G., Barros, A., Silva, B., Belém, L., Ferreira, V., Fonseca, A., Castro, P., Santos, T., Lemos, T. and Hérickson, W., 2020. Cold-water immersion does not accelerate performance recovery after 10-km street run: Randomized controlled clinical trial. *Research Quarterly for Exercise and Sport, 91*(2), pp. 228–238.

Dębski, P., Białas, E. and Gnat, R., 2019. The parameters of foam rolling, self-myofascial release treatment: A review of the literature. *Biomedical Human Kinetics, 11*(1), pp. 36–46.

de Freitas, V.H., Ramos, S.P., Bara-Filho, M.G., Freitas, D.G., Coimbra, D.R., Cecchini, R., Guarnier, F.A. and Nakamura, F.Y., 2019. Effect of cold-water immersion performed on successive days on physical performance, muscle damage, and inflammatory, hormonal, and oxidative stress markers in volleyball players. *The Journal of Strength & Conditioning Research, 33*(2), pp. 502–513.

Demirhan, B., Yaman, M., Cengiz, A., Saritas, N. and Günay, M., 2015. Comparison of ice massage versus cold-water immersion on muscle damage and DOMS levels of elite wrestlers. *The Anthropologist, 19*(1), pp. 123–129.

Dunning, J., Butts, R., Mourad, F., Young, I., Flannagan, S. and Perreault, T. 2014. Dry needling: a literature review with implications for clinical practice guidelines. *Physical Therapy Reviews: PTR, 19*(4), pp. 252–265.

DuPont, W.H., Meuris, B.J., Hardesty, V.H., Barnhart, E.C., Tompkins, L.H., Golden, M.J., Usher, C.J., Spence, P.A., Caldwell, L.K., Post, E.M. and Beeler, M.K., 2017. The effects combining cryo-compression therapy following an acute bout of resistance exercise on performance and recovery. *Journal of Sports Science & Medicine, 16*(3), p. 333.

Engel, F., Stockinger, C., Woll, A. and Sperlich, B., 2016. Effects of compression garments on performance and recovery in endurance athletes. In: Engel, F. and Sperlich, B. (eds.), *Compression garments in sports: Athletic performance and recovery* (pp. 33–61). Cham: Springer. doi: 10.1007/978-3-319-39480-0_2

Fernández-Carnero, J., La Touche, R., Ortega-Santiago, R., Galan-del-Rio, F., Pesquera, J., Ge, H.Y. and Fernández-de-Las-Peñas, C., 2010. Short-term effects of dry needling of active myofascial trigger points in the masseter muscle in patients with temporomandibular disorders. *Journal of Orofacial Pain, 24*(1), pp. 106–112. PMID: 20213036.

France, S., Bown, J., Nowosilskyj, M., Mott, M., Rand, S. and Walters, J., 2014. Evidence for the use of dry needling and physiotherapy in the management of cervicogenic or tension-type headache: A systematic review. *Cephalalgia, 34*(12), pp. 994–1003.

Freire, B., Geremia, J., Baroni, B.M. and Vaz, M.A., 2016. Effects of cryotherapy methods on circulatory, metabolic, inflammatory and neural properties: A systematic review. *Fisioterapia em Movimento, 29*(2), pp. 389–398.

Gattie, E., Cleland, J.A. and Snodgrass, S., 2017. The effectiveness of trigger point dry needling for musculoskeletal conditions by physical therapists: A systematic review and meta-analysis. *Journal of Orthopaedic & Sports Physical Therapy, 47*(3), pp. 133–149.

Gerber, L.H., Shah, J., Rosenberger, W., Armstrong, K., Turo, D., Otto, P., Heimur, J., Thaker, N. and Sikdar, S., 2015. Dry needling alters trigger points in the upper trapezius muscle and reduces pain in subjects with chronic myofascial pain. *PM&R, 7*(7), pp. 711–718.

Govus, A.D., Andersson, E.P., Shannon, O.M., Provis, H., Karlsson, M. and McGawley, K., 2018. Commercially available compression garments or electrical stimulation do not enhance recovery following a sprint competition in elite cross-country skiers. *European Journal of Sport Science, 18*(10), pp. 1299–1308.

Grainger, A., Comfort, P. and Heffernan, S., 2020. No effect of partial-body cryotherapy on restoration of countermovement jump or well-being performance in elite rugby union players during the competitive phase of the season. *International Journal of Sports Physiology and Performance, 15*(1), pp. 98–104.

Gulick, D.T., 2018. Instrument-assisted soft tissue mobilization increases myofascial trigger point pain threshold. *Journal of Bodywork and Movement Therapies, 22*(2), pp. 341–345.

Gutiérrez-Rojas, C., González, I., Navarrete, E., Olivares, E., Rojas, J., Tordecilla, D. and Bustamante, C., 2015. The effect of combining myofascial release with ice application on a latent trigger point in the forearm of young adults: a randomized clinical trial. *Myopain, 23*(3–4), pp. 201–208.

Hall, M.L., Mackie, A.C. and Ribeiro, D.C., 2018. Effects of dry needling trigger point therapy in the shoulder region on patients with upper extremity pain and dysfunction: A systematic review with meta-analysis. *Physiotherapy, 104*(2), pp. 167–177.

Halperin, I., Aboodarda, S.J., Button, D.C., Andersen, L.L. and Behm, D.G., 2014. Roller massager improves range of motion of plantar flexor muscles without subsequent decreases in force parameters. *International Journal of Sports Physical Therapy, 9*(1), p. 92.

Hammer, W.I. and Pfefer, M.T., 2005. Treatment of a case of subacute lumbar compartment syndrome using the Graston technique. *Journal of Manipulative and Physiological Therapeutics, 28*(3), pp. 199–204.

Healey, K.C., Hatfield, D.L., Blanpied, P., Dorfman, L.R. and Riebe, D., 2014. The effects of myofascial release with foam rolling on performance. *The Journal of Strength & Conditioning Research, 28*(1), pp. 61–68.

Hendricks, S., den Hollander, S., Lombard, W. and Parker, R., 2019. Effects of foam rolling on performance and recovery: A systematic review of the literature to guide practitioners on the use of foam rolling. *Journal of Bodywork and Movement Therapies.*

Higgins, T.R., Greene, D.A. and Baker, M.K., 2017. Effects of cold-water immersion and contrast water therapy for recovery from team sport: a systematic review and meta-analysis. *The Journal of Strength & Conditioning Research, 31*(5), pp. 1443–1460.

Hodgson, D.D., Lima, C.D., Low, J.L. and Behm, D.G., 2018. Four weeks of roller massage training did not impact range of motion, pain pressure threshold, voluntary contractile properties or jump performance. *International Journal of Sports Physical Therapy, 13*(5), p. 835.

Hohenauer, E., Taeymans, J., Baeyens, J.P., Clarys, P. and Clijsen, R., 2015. The effect of post-exercise cryotherapy on recovery characteristics: A systematic review and meta-analysis. *PLoS One, 10*(9), p. e0139028.

Hohenauer, E., Costello, J.T., Stoop, R., Küng, U.M., Clarys, P., Deliens, T. and Clijsen, R., 2018. Cold-water or partial-body cryotherapy? Comparison of physiological responses and recovery following muscle damage. *Scandinavian Journal of Medicine & Science in Sports, 28*(3), pp. 1252–1262.

Hotfiel, T., Swoboda, B., Krinner, S., Grim, C., Engelhardt, M., Uder, M. and Heiss, R.U., 2017. Acute effects of lateral thigh foam rolling on arterial tissue perfusion determined by spectral Doppler and power Doppler ultrasound. *Journal of Strength and Conditioning Research, 31*(4), pp. 893–900.

Howatson, G., Gaze, D. and Van Someren, K.A., 2005. The efficacy of ice massage in the treatment of exercise-induced muscle damage. *Scandinavian Journal of Medicine & Science in Sports, 15*(6), pp. 416–422.

Hsieh, Y.L., Kao, M.J., Kuan, T.S., Chen, S.M., Chen, J.T. and Hong, C.Z., 2007. Dry needling to a key myofascial trigger point may reduce the irritability of satellite MTrPs. *American Journal of Physical Medicine & Rehabilitation, 86*(5), pp. 397–403.

Hu, H.T., Gao, H., Ma, R.J., Zhao, X.F., Tian, H.F. and Li, L., 2018. Is dry needling effective for low back pain? A systematic review and PRISMA-compliant meta-analysis. *Medicine, 97*(26), p. e11225. https://doi.org/10.1097/MD.0000000000011225

Ihsan, M., Watson, G. and Abbiss, C.R., 2016. What are the physiological mechanisms for post-exercise cold water immersion in the recovery from prolonged endurance and intermittent exercise? *Sports Medicine, 46*(8), pp. 1095–1109.

Ikeda, N., Otsuka, S., Kawanishi, Y. and Kawakami, Y., 2019. Effects of instrument-assisted soft tissue mobilization on musculoskeletal properties. *Medicine and Science in Sports and Exercise, 51*(10), p. 2166.

Jackson, M.D., Rowe, K. and Davenport, T.E., 2016. Trigger point dry needling for musculoskeletal pain and disability: A systematic review of comparative effectiveness research. *Orthopaedic Physical Therapy Practice, 28*(3), p. 178.

Jay, K., Sundstrup, E., Søndergaard, S.D., Behm, D., Brandt, M., Særvoll, C.A., Jakobsen, M.D. and Andersen, L.L., 2014. Specific and cross over effects of massage for muscle soreness: Randomized controlled trial. *International Journal of Sports Physical Therapy, 9*(1), p. 82.

Junker, D.H. and Stöggl, T.L., 2015. The foam roll as a tool to improve hamstring flexibility. *The Journal of Strength & Conditioning Research*, 29(12), pp. 3480–3485.

Kamali, F., Mohamadi, M., Fakheri, L. and Mohammadnejad, F., 2019. Dry needling versus friction massage to treat tension type headache: A randomized clinical trial. *Journal of Bodywork and Movement Therapies*, 23(1), pp. 89–93.

Kelly, S. and Beardsley, C., 2016. Specific and cross-over effects of foam rolling on ankle dorsiflexion range of motion. *International Journal of Sports Physical Therapy*, 11(4), p. 544.

Khoshnevis, S., Craik, N.K. and Diller, K.R., 2015. Cold-induced vasoconstriction may persist long after cooling ends: An evaluation of multiple cryotherapy units. *Knee Surgery, Sports Traumatology, Arthroscopy*, 23(9), pp. 2475–2483.

Kim, K., Kuang, S., Song, Q., Gavin, T.P. and Roseguini, B.T., 2019. Impact of heat therapy on recovery after eccentric exercise in humans. *Journal of Applied Physiology*, 126(4), pp. 965–976.

Kim, J.I., Lee, M.S., Lee, D.H., Boddy, K. and Ernst, E., 2009. Cupping for treating pain: a systematic review. *Evidence-Based Complementary and Alternative Medicine*, 2011. doi: 10.1093/ecam/nep035

Kim, J., Sung, D.J. and Lee, J., 2017. Therapeutic effectiveness of instrument-assisted soft tissue mobilization for soft tissue injury: Mechanisms and practical application. *Journal of Exercise Rehabilitation*, 13(1), p. 12.

Laffaye, G., Torrinha Da Silva, D. and Delafontaine, A., 2019. Self-myofascial release effect with foam rolling on recovery after high-intensity interval training. *Frontiers in Physiology*, 10, p. 1287.

Laudner, K., Compton, B.D., McLoda, T.A. and Walters, C.M., 2014. Acute effects of instrument assisted soft tissue mobilization for improving posterior shoulder range of motion in collegiate baseball players. *International Journal of Sports Physical Therapy*, 9(1), p. 1.

Lavelle, E.D., Lavelle, W. and Smith, H.S., 2007. Myofascial trigger points. *Anesthesiology Clinics*, 25(4), pp. 841–851.

Lederer, A.K., Maly, C., Weinert, T. and Huber, R., 2019. Tissue stiffness is not related to pain experience: An individually controlled study in patients with chronic neck and back pain. *Evidence-Based Complementary and Alternative Medicine*, 2019, p. 1907168. https://doi.org/10.1155/2019/1907168

Lee, J., Young, A., Erb, N.J. and Herzog, V.W., 2020. Acute and residual effects of IASTM and roller massage stick on hamstring range of motion. *Journal of Allied Health*, 49(1), pp. 51E–55E.

Leeder, J.D., Van Someren, K.A., Bell, P.G., Spence, J.R., Jewell, A.P., Gaze, D. and Howatson, G., 2015. Effects of seated and standing cold water immersion on recovery from repeated sprinting. *Journal of Sports Sciences*, 33(15), pp. 1544–1552.

Leeder, J.D., Godfrey, M., Gibbon, D., Gaze, D., Davison, G.W., Van Someren, K.A. and Howatson, G., 2019. Cold water immersion improves recovery of sprint speed following a simulated tournament. *European Journal of Sport Science*, 19(9), pp. 1166–1174.

Liu, L., Huang, Q.M., Liu, Q.G., Ye, G., Bo, C.Z., Chen, M.J. and Li, P., 2015. Effectiveness of dry needling for myofascial trigger points associated with neck and shoulder pain: A systematic review and meta-analysis. *Archives of Physical Medicine and Rehabilitation*, 96(5), pp. 944–955.

Lyu, B.J., Lee, C.L., Chang, W.D. and Chang, N.J., 2020. Effects of vibration rolling with and without dynamic muscle contraction on ankle range of motion, proprioception, muscle strength and agility in young adults: A crossover study. *International Journal of Environmental Research and Public Health*, 17(1), p. 354.

MacDonald, G.Z., 2013. Foam rolling as a recovery tool following an intense bout of physical activity. Doctoral dissertation, Memorial University of Newfoundland.

MacDonald, G.Z., Penney, M.D., Mullaley, M.E., Cuconato, A.L., Drake, C.D., Behm, D.G. and Button, D.C., 2013. An acute bout of self-myofascial release increases range of motion without a subsequent decrease in muscle activation or force. *The Journal of Strength & Conditioning Research*, 27(3), pp. 812–821.

MacDonald, N., Baker, R. and Cheatham, S.W., 2016. The effects of instrument assisted soft tissue mobilization on lower extremity muscle performance: A randomized controlled trial. *International Journal of Sports Physical Therapy*, 11(7), p. 1040.

Machado, A.F., Ferreira, P.H., Micheletti, J.K., de Almeida, A.C., Lemes, Í.R., Vanderlei, F.M., Junior, J.N. and Pastre, C.M., 2016. Can water temperature and immersion time influence the effect of cold-water immersion on muscle soreness? A systematic review and meta-analysis. *Sports Medicine*, 46(4), pp. 503–514.

Madoni, S.N., Costa, P.B., Coburn, J.W. and Galpin, A.J., 2018. Effects of foam rolling on range of motion, peak torque, muscle activation, and the hamstrings-to-quadriceps strength ratios. *The Journal of Strength & Conditioning Research*, 32(7), pp. 1821–1830.

Markovic, G., 2015. Acute effects of instrument assisted soft tissue mobilization vs. foam rolling on knee and hip range of motion in soccer players. *Journal of Bodywork and Movement Therapies*, 19(4), pp. 690–696.

Marqués-Jiménez, D., Calleja-González, J., Arratibel, I., Delextrat, A. and Terrados, N., 2016. Are compression garments effective for the recovery of exercise-induced muscle damage? A systematic review with meta-analysis. *Physiology & Behavior*, 153, pp. 133–148.

Marques-Jimenez, D., Calleja-González, J., Arratibel, I., Delextrat, A., Uriarte, F. and Terrados, N., 2018. Physiological and physical responses to wearing compression garments during soccer matches and recovery. *The Journal of Sports Medicine and Physical Fitness*, 58(11), pp. 1642–1651.

Masuda, A., Koga, Y., Hattanmaru, M., Minagoe, S. and Tei, C., 2005. The effects of repeated thermal therapy for patients with chronic pain. *Psychotherapy and Psychosomatics*, 74(5), pp. 288–294.

Mayer, J.M., Ralph, L., Look, M., Erasala, G.N., Verna, J.L., Matheson, L.N. and Mooney, V., 2005. Treating acute low back pain with continuous low-level heat wrap therapy and/or exercise: A randomized controlled trial. *The Spine Journal*, 5(4), pp. 395–403.

Mohr, A.R., Long, B.C. and Goad, C.L., 2014. Effect of foam rolling and static stretching on passive hip-flexion range of motion. *Journal of Sport Rehabilitation*, 23(4), pp. 296–299.

Monteiro, E.R., Vigotsky, A.D., da Silva Novaes, J. and Škarabot, J., 2018. Acute effects of different anterior thigh self-massage on hip range-of-motion in trained men. *International Journal of Sports Physical Therapy*, 13(1), p. 104.

Monteiro, E.R., da Silva Novaes, J., Cavanaugh, M.T., Hoogenboom, B.J., Steele, J., Vingren, J.L. and Škarabot, J., 2019. Quadriceps foam rolling and rolling massage increases hip flexion and extension passive range-of-motion. *Journal of Bodywork and Movement Therapies*, 23(3), pp. 575–580.

Morihisa, R., Eskew, J., McNamara, A. and Young, J., 2016. Dry needling in subjects with muscular trigger points in the lower quarter: A systematic review. *International Journal of Sports Physical Therapy*, 11(1), p. 1.

Moura, C.D.C., Chaves, É.D.C.L., Cardoso, A.C.L.R., Nogueira, D.A., Corrêa, H.P. and Chianca, T.C.M., 2018. Cupping therapy and chronic back pain: Systematic review and meta-analysis. *Revista latino-americana de enfermagem*, 26, p. e3094. doi: 10.1590/1518-8345.2888.3094

Murray, A.M., Jones, T.W., Horobeanu, C., Turner, A.P. and Sproule, J., 2016. Sixty seconds of foam rolling does not affect functional flexibility or change muscle temperature in adolescent athletes. *International Journal of Sports Physical Therapy*, 11(5), p. 765.

Nadler, S.F., Steiner, D.J., Erasala, G.N., Hengehold, D.A., Hinkle, R.T., Goodale, M.B., Abeln, S.B. and Weingand, K.W., 2002. Continuous low-level heat wrap therapy provides more efficacy than Ibuprofen and acetaminophen for acute low back pain. *Spine*, 27(10), pp. 1012–1017.

Nadler, S.F., Weingand, K. and Kruse, R.J., 2004. The physiologic basis and clinical applications of cryotherapy and thermotherapy for the pain practitioner. *Pain Physician*, 7(3), pp. 395–400.

Okamoto, T., Masuhara, M. and Ikuta, K., 2014. Acute effects of self-myofascial release using a foam roller on arterial function. *The Journal of Strength & Conditioning Research*, 28(1), pp. 69–73.

Ong, J. and Claydon, L.S., 2014. The effect of dry needling for myofascial trigger points in the neck and shoulders: A systematic review and meta-analysis. *Journal of Bodywork and Movement Therapies*, *18*(3), pp. 390–398.

Paz, G.A., Maia, M.F., Santana, H., Silva, J.B. and Lima, V.P., 2017. Electromyographic analysis of muscles activation during sit-and-reach test adopting self-myofascial release with foam rolling versus traditional warm up. *Journal of Athletic Enhancement 6: 1 of 4*, pp. 26–28.

Peacock, C.A., Krein, D.D., Antonio, J., Sanders, G.J., Silver, T.A. and Colas, M., 2015. Comparing acute bouts of sagittal plane progression foam rolling vs. frontal plane progression foam rolling. *The Journal of Strength & Conditioning Research*, *29*(8), pp. 2310–2315.

Peake, J.M., Roberts, L.A., Figueiredo, V.C., Egner, I., Krog, S., Aas, S.N., Suzuki, K., Markworth, J.F., Coombes, J.S., Cameron-Smith, D. and Raastad, T., 2017. The effects of cold-water immersion and active recovery on inflammation and cell stress responses in human skeletal muscle after resistance exercise. *The Journal of Physiology*, *595*(3), pp. 695–711.

Pearcey, G.E., Bradbury-Squires, D.J., Kawamoto, J.E., Drinkwater, E.J., Behm, D.G. and Button, D.C., 2015. Foam rolling for delayed-onset muscle soreness and recovery of dynamic performance measures. *Journal of Athletic Training*, *50*(1), pp. 5–13.

Pelana, R., Maulana, A., Winata, B., Widiastuti, W., Sukur, A., Kuswahyudi, K., Juriana, J. and Hermawan, R., 2019. Effect of contrast water therapy on blood lactate concentration after high-intensity interval training in elite futsal players. *Physiotherapy Quarterly*, *27*(3), pp. 12–19.

Perrcault, T., Dunning, J. and Butts, R., 2017. The local twitch response during trigger point dry needling: Is it necessary for successful outcomes? *Journal of Bodywork and Movement Therapies*, *21*(4), pp. 940–947.

Petrofsky, J., Berk, L., Bains, G., Khowailed, I.A., Lee, H. and Laymon, M., 2017. The efficacy of sustained heat treatment on delayed-onset muscle soreness. *Clinical Journal of Sport Medicine*, *27*(4), pp. 329–337.

Portillo-Soto, A., Eberman, L.E., Demchak, T.J. and Peebles, C., 2014. Comparison of blood flow changes with soft tissue mobilization and massage therapy. *The Journal of Alternative and Complementary Medicine*, *20*(12), pp. 932–936.

Putra, A.Y., Setijono, H. and Mintarto, E., 2020. The difference effect of recovery in warm water and aroma therapy Sauna recovery against decreased lactic acid levels after submaximal physical activity. *Britain International of Humanities and Social Sciences (BIoHS) Journal*, *2*(1), pp. 256–263.

Qu, C., Wu, Z., Xu, M., Qin, F., Dong, Y., Wang, Z. and Zhao, J., 2020. Cryotherapy models and timing-sequence recovery of exercise-induced muscle damage in middle-and long-distance runners. *Journal of Athletic Training*, *55*(4), pp. 329–335.

Rey, E., Padrón-Cabo, A., Costa, P.B. and Barcala-Furelos, R., 2019. Effects of foam rolling as a recovery tool in professional soccer players. *The Journal of Strength & Conditioning Research*, *33*(8), pp. 2194–2201.

Richman, E.D., Tyo, B.M. and Nicks, C.R., 2019. Combined effects of self-myofascial release and dynamic stretching on range of motion, jump, sprint, and agility performance. *The Journal of Strength & Conditioning Research*, *33*(7), pp. 1795–1803.

Romero-Moraleda, B., La Touche, R., Lerma-Lara, S., Ferrer-Peña, R., Paredes, V., Peinado, A.B. and Muñoz-García, D., 2017. Neurodynamic mobilization and foam rolling improved delayed-onset muscle soreness in a healthy adult population: a randomized controlled clinical trial. *Peer J*, *5*, p. e3908.

Rose, C., Edwards, K.M., Siegler, J., Graham, K. and Caillaud, C., 2017. Whole-body cryotherapy as a recovery technique after exercise: A review of the literature. *International Journal of Sports Medicine*, *38*(14), pp. 1049–1060.

Roylance, D.S., George, J.D., Hammer, A.M., Rencher, N., Fellingham, G.W., Hager, R.L. and Myrer, W.J., 2013. Evaluating acute changes in joint range-of-motion using self-myofascial release, postural alignment exercises, and static stretches. *International Journal of Exercise Science*, *6*(4), p. 6.

Saini, D., 2015. Cryotherapy – an inevitable part of sports medicine and its benefits for sport injury. *IJAR*, *1*(4), pp. 324–327.

Schafer, M.D., Tom, J.C., Girouard, T.J., Navalta, J.W., Turner, C.L. and Radzak, K.N., 2020. Cupping therapy does not influence healthy adult's hamstring range of motion compared to control or sham conditions. *International Journal of Exercise Science*, 13(3), p. 216.

Schleip R., 2003. Fascial plasticity – a new neurobiological explanation: Part 1. *Journal of Bodywork and Movement Therapies*, 1;7(1), pp. 11–19.

Schleip, R. and Müller, D.G., 2013. Training principles for fascial connective tissues: Scientific foundation and suggested practical applications. *Journal of Bodywork and Movement Therapies*, 17(1), pp. 103–115.

Seco-Calvo, J., Mielgo-Ayuso, J., Calvo-Lobo, C. and Córdova, A., 2020. Cold water immersion as a strategy for muscle recovery in professional basketball players during the competitive season. *Journal of Sport Rehabilitation*, 29(3), pp. 301–309.

Seffrin, C.B., Cattano, N.M., Reed, M.A. and Gardiner-Shires, A.M., 2019. Instrument-Assisted soft tissue mobilization: A systematic review and effect-size analysis. *Journal of Athletic Training*, 54(7), pp. 808–821.

Škarabot, J., Beardsley, C. and Štirn, I., 2015. Comparing the effects of self-myofascial release with static stretching on ankle range-of-motion in adolescent athletes. *International Journal of Sports Physical Therapy*, 10(2), p. 203.

Skinner, B., Moss, R. and Hammond, L., 2020. A systematic review and meta-analysis of the effects of foam rolling on range of motion, recovery and markers of athletic performance. *Journal of Bodywork and Movement Therapies*, 24(3), pp. 105–122.

Skorski, S., Schimpchen, J., Pfeiffer, M., Ferrauti, A., Kellmann, M. and Meyer, T., 2019. Effects of postexercise Sauna bathing on recovery of swim performance. *International Journal of Sports Physiology and Performance*, 1(aop), pp. 1–7.

Sterling, M., Vicenzino, B., Souvlis, T. and Connelly, L.B., 2015. Dry-needling and exercise for chronic whiplash-associated disorders: A randomized single-blind placebo-controlled trial. *Pain*, 156(4), pp. 635–643.

Stroiney, D.A., Mokris, R.L., Hanna, G.R. and Ranney, J.D., 2020. Examination of self-myofascial release vs. instrument-assisted soft-tissue mobilization techniques on vertical and horizontal power in recreational athletes. *The Journal of Strength & Conditioning Research*, 34(1), pp. 79–88.

Su, H., Chang, N.J., Wu, W.L., Guo, L.Y. and Chu, I.H., 2017. Acute effects of foam rolling, static stretching, and dynamic stretching during warm-ups on muscular flexibility and strength in young adults. *Journal of Sport Rehabilitation*, 26(6), pp. 469–477.

Sullivan, K.M., Silvey, D.B., Button, D.C. and Behm, D.G., 2013. Roller-massager application to the hamstrings increases sit-and-reach range of motion within five to ten seconds without performance impairments. *International Journal of Sports Physical Therapy*, 8(3), p. 228.

Threlkeld, A.J., 1992. The effects of manual therapy on connective tissue. *Physical Therapy*, 72(12), pp. 893–902.

Vaile, J.M., Gill, N.D. and Blazevich, A.J., 2007. The effect of contrast water therapy on symptoms of delayed onset muscle soreness. *The Journal of Strength & Conditioning Research*, 21(3), pp. 697–702.

Vardiman, J.P., Siedlik, J., Herda, T., Hawkins, W., Cooper, M., Graham, Z.A., Deckert, J. and Gallagher, P., 2015. Instrument-assisted soft tissue mobilization: effects on the properties of human plantar flexors. *International Journal of Sports Medicine*, 36(03), pp. 197–203.

Vier, C., de Almeida, M.B., Neves, M.L., dos Santos, A.R.S. and Bracht, M.A., 2019. The effectiveness of dry needling for patients with orofacial pain associated with temporomandibular dysfunction: A systematic review and meta-analysis. *Brazilian Journal of Physical Therapy*, 23(1), pp. 3–11.

Vigotsky, A.D., Lehman, G.J., Contreras, B., Beardsley, C., Chung, B. and Feser, E.H., 2015. Acute effects of anterior thigh foam rolling on hip angle, knee angle, and rectus femoris length in the modified Thomas test. *PeerJ*, 3, p. e1281.

Volpato, M.P., Breda, I.C., de Carvalho, R.C., de Castro Moura, C., Ferreira, L.L., Silva, M.L. and Silva, J.R., 2020. Single cupping therapy session improves pain, sleep, and disability in patients with nonspecific chronic low back pain. *Journal of Acupuncture and Meridian Studies*, 13(2), pp. 48–52.

Wiewelhove, T., Döweling, A., Schneider, C., Hottenrott, L., Meyer, T., Kellmann, M., Pfeiffer, M. and Ferrauti, A., 2019. A meta-analysis of the effects of foam rolling on performance and recovery. *Frontiers in Physiology*, *10*, p. 376.

Wilcock, I.M., Cronin, J.B. and Hing, W.A., 2006. Physiological response to water immersion. *Sports Medicine*, *36*(9), pp. 747–765.

Wilke, J., Mueller, A.L., Giesche, F., Power, G., Ahmedi, H. and Behm, D.G., 2020. Acute effects of foam rolling on range of motion in healthy adults: a systematic review with multilevel meta-analysis. *Sports Medicine*, *50*(2), pp. 387–402.

Williams, J.G., Gard, H.I., Gregory, J.M., Gibson, A. and Austin, J., 2019. The Effects of Cupping on Hamstring Flexibility in College Soccer Players. *Journal of Sport Rehabilitation*, *28*(4), pp. 350–353.

Wilson, L.J., Dimitriou, L., Hills, F.A., Gondek, M.B. and Cockburn, E., 2019. Whole body cryotherapy, cold water immersion, or a placebo following resistance exercise: A case of mind over matter? *European Journal of Applied Physiology*, *119*(1), pp. 135–147.

Ziaeifar, M., Arab, A.M., Karimi, N. and Nourbakhsh, M.R., 2014. The effect of dry needling on pain, pressure pain threshold and disability in patients with a myofascial trigger point in the upper trapezius muscle. *Journal of Bodywork and Movement Therapies*, *18*(2), pp. 298–305.

Conclusion

Sports performance massage aims to inform the student, the athlete, and practising therapist how to use scientific evidence to inform their practice when working with athletic populations. Athletes frequently ask how they can recover as quickly as possible from fatigue, heal from injury and improve their subsequent performances. This book will empower the therapist by giving them greater confidence, increase their scientific awareness and improve their critical thinking.

An extensive search of the literature appears to indicate that massage prior to athletic performance or in conjunction with an active warm up routine could have effects on athletic performance ranging from detrimental (Arabaci, 2008; Arazi et al., 2012) to mixed, (Fletcher, 2010; Arroyo-Morrales et al., 2011), or neutral (Goodwin et al., 2007; McKechnie et al., 2007; Bedford & Robbins, 2016; Bedford et al., 2018) especially in jumping and sprinting activities. In addition, as massage stimulates sensory afferent fibres in the skin (Sarli & Agus, 2014), therefore, receiving a massage pre-event may provide some short-term pain relief.

Furthermore, a number of other studies have reported beneficial outcomes on perceived fatigue (Szabo et al., 2008; Jooste et al., 2013; Nunes et al., 2016), tightness, and perceptions of tightness and fatigue, therefore massage as a treatment should not be overlooked. Zusman (2013) found that positive communication, such as "now I will give you treatment and it will reduce your pain" could generate positive expectations, making it unclear whether the effects of massage are physiological or in fact psychological when effectively measuring perceived amounts of pain or discomfort. It should also be remembered that the hands are the sensors that evaluate skin temperature, moisture and texture, the quality of the underlying subcutaneous tissue, muscles, fascia and the position of bony landmarks, and are used to guide movement in assessment of quality and range of motion (Kidd, 2009).

A number of articles found that massage and foam rolling have a positive effect on delayed onset muscle soreness (DOMS). For example, Visconti et al. (2015) found DOMS responds to massage but does not appear to respond to other modalities such as rest, suggesting that an intervention that results in repeated stimulation of afferent nerve endings and nociceptors creates an analgesic response. Other positive effects on foam rolling and the reduction of delayed onset muscle soreness have also been noted by Jay et al. (2014), Pearcey et al. (2015), and Romero-Moraleda et al. (2017), although the majority of massage and foam rolling investigations rely on subjective markers. The results from massage and foam rolling (self-myofascial release) studies are difficult to interpret, as the pressure used, rate (speed) at which techniques are performed, duration of treatment and protocols used are either not reported, poorly described, or biased. However, it does appear that both massage and foam rolling do assist in relieving the symptoms of delayed onset muscle soreness.

Cryotherapy is another modality frequently used as a post-exercise recovery intervention to relieve pain, reduce muscle spasm and reduce the effects of delayed onset muscle soreness. However, the temperature of the water, length of time and depth submerged still remain controversial. This was noted in Rose et al.'s (2017) review of the literature on whole-body cryotherapy (WBC) as a recovery technique after exercise. The authors commented that study designs were vastly different, making inferences difficult. However, they did conclude from their review that WBC may be successful in enhancing maximal voluntary contractions (MVC) and returning athletes to pre-exercise strength at a faster rate, with WBC treatment conditions recording pain scores on average 31% lower than control groups. However, other authors have disagreed about its effectiveness, including Costello and colleagues (2016), Wilson et al. (2019), and Krueger et al. (2019). To this end, it appears whole body cryotherapy (more so than cold-water immersion [CWI]) may have a positive effect for some individuals on both physiological and psychological (placebo effect) recovery markers, possibly due to inconsistent timings, water depths, and temperatures recorded in the cold-water immersion trials.

Petrissage techniques involve the rhymical lifting and squeezing of muscles, so it is easy to see a link with compression garments. Lee et al. (2021) concluded that wearing compression garments during passive recovery from exercise seems to be beneficial for performance recovery and DOMS. However, other findings were not so positive, including a study of 55 articles involving 788 participants discussed in a review by Engel et al. (2016). Govus et al. (2018) concurred, finding that neither compression garments nor neuromuscular electrical stimulation promoted physiological or perceptual recovery compared with a control group.

Although not covered on the sports massage syllabus, cupping, instrument-assisted soft tissue massage (fascial abrasion) and dry needling are frequently used by therapists alongside traditional sports massage techniques, although the justification for their use is mixed. For example, in a systematic review addressing the effects of cupping for treating pain, Kim et al. (2011) suggested that there was evidence for the effectiveness of cupping in the management of pain conditions. However, the total number of randomised controlled trials ($n = 7$) included in their analysis and the methodological quality were too low to draw firm conclusions. Bridgett et al. (2018) agreed, noting that the majority of the studies in their review had an unclear or high risk of bias. Arias-Buria et al. (2020) and Gerber et al. (2015) concluded that dry needling could be recommended for treating trigger points and have shown to reduce pain and change myofascial trigger point status. Meanwhile, Gattie et al. (2017) suggested there was very low- to moderate-quality evidence that dry needling is more effective than no treatment, sham dry needling, and other treatments for reducing pain and improving pressure pain threshold in patients presenting with musculoskeletal pain. In light of this, it appears that the use of cupping is not yet warranted, although dry needling may assist in the reduction of trigger points.

Fascial abrasion or instrument-assisted soft tissue massage (IASTM) uses a stainless steel concave and convex instrument which makes it easier to apply pressure over a smaller surface area, allowing the therapist to focus on more specific areas during treatment. Cheatham et al.'s (2016) systematic review of 7 articles revealed that the majority of articles has indicated insignificant results which challenges the efficacy of IASTM as a treatment for common musculoskeletal pathology, which may be due to the methodological variability among studies, however, there appears to be some evidence supporting its ability to increase short term joint ROM.

Kim et al. (2017) summarised, published articles consisting mostly of case reports rather than experimental studies, with some of the case reports failing to present the details of the IASTM protocol that was applied, make results difficult to interpret. As fascial abrasion involves scraping the instrument over the skin, there is likely to be a counter-irritation with an accompanying local analgesic effect, including local blood perfusion. Therefore, the use of fascial abrasion techniques may have a short-term benefit on pain relief.

In summary, the use of massage, foam rolling, compression garments, dry needling and whole-body cryotherapy all appear to provide some relief from muscular soreness post-exercise. Pre-performance massage, foam rolling and stretching are unlikely to be detrimental to performance, especially if they are of a short duration and form part of a general active warm-up routine. It is unlikely that pre-performance massage and stretching provide any performance benefit physiologically aside from short-term pain relief (massage). Time spent with an athlete prior to, or following, training or competition may be more valuable psychologically than physiologically, so these treatment modalities should not be dismissed. Continued research on massage, foam rolling and other modalities with standardised protocols is warranted, with specific attention to depth of pressure, the time-course effect and time of administration pre- and post-performance requiring investigation in well-conducted trials before firm conclusions can be drawn.

References

Arabaci, R., 2008. Acute effects of pre-event lower limb massage on explosive and high-speed motor capacities and flexibility. *Journal of Sports Science & Medicine*, 7(4), p. 549.

Arazi, H., Asadi, A. and Hoseini, K., 2012. Comparison of two different warm-ups (static-stretching and massage): Effects on flexibility and explosive power. *Acta Kinesiologica*, 6(1), pp. 55–59.

Arias-Buría, J.L., Monroy-Acevedo, Á., Fernández-de-Las-Peñas, C., Gallego-Sendarrubias, G.M., Ortega-Santiago, R. and Plaza-Manzano, G., 2020. Effects of dry needling of active trigger points in the scalene muscles in individuals with mechanical neck pain: A randomized clinical trial. *Acupuncture in Medicine*, 38(6), pp. 380–387.

Arroyo-Morales, M., Fernández-Lao, C., Ariza-García, A., Toro-Velasco, C., Winters, M., Díaz-Rodríguez, L., Cantarero-Villanueva, I., Huijbregts, P. and Fernández-De-las-Peñas, C., 2011. Psychophysiological effects of preperformance massage before isokinetic exercise. *The Journal of Strength & Conditioning Research*, 25(2), pp. 481–488.

Bedford, S. and Robbins, D., 2016. The acute effects of massage are not detrimental to grip strength in sub-elite racquet players. *Medicine & Science in Tennis*, 21(1), pp. 24–27.

Bedford, S., Robbins, D. and Fletcher, I., 2018. Effects of an active warm up and warm up massage on agility, perceived exertion and flexibility in tennis players. *Journal of Science and Medicine in Tennis*, 23(2), pp. 16–22.

Bridgett, R., Klose, P., Duffield, R., Mydock, S. and Lauche, R., 2018. Effects of cupping therapy in amateur and professional athletes: Systematic review of randomized controlled trials. *The Journal of Alternative and Complementary Medicine*, 24(3), pp. 208–219.

Cheatham, S.W., Lee, M., Cain, M. and Baker, R., 2016. The efficacy of instrument assisted soft tissue mobilization: A systematic review. *The Journal of the Canadian Chiropractic Association*, 60(3), p. 200.

Costello, J.T., Baker, P.R., Minett, G.M., Bieuzen, F., Stewart, I.B. and Bleakley, C., 2016. Cochrane review: Whole-body cryotherapy (extreme cold air exposure) for preventing and treating muscle soreness after exercise in adults. *Journal of Evidence-Based Medicine*, 9(1), pp. 43–44.

Engel, F., Stockinger, C., Woll, A. and Sperlich, B., 2016. Effects of compression garments on performance and recovery in endurance athletes. In F. Engel and B. Sperlich (eds). *Compression Garments in Sports: Athletic Performance and Recovery* (pp. 33–61). Springer, Cham.

Fletcher, I.M., 2010. The effects of precompetition massage on the kinematic parameters of 20-m sprint performance. *The Journal of Strength & Conditioning Research*, 24(5), pp. 1179–1183.

Gattie, E., Cleland, J.A. and Snodgrass, S., 2017. The effectiveness of trigger point dry needling for musculoskeletal conditions by physical therapists: A systematic review and meta-analysis. *Journal of Orthopaedic & Sports Physical Therapy*, 47(3), pp. 133–149.

Gerber, L.H., Shah, J., Rosenberger, W., Armstrong, K., Turo, D., Otto, P., Heimur, J., Thaker, N. and Sikdar, S., 2015. Dry needling alters trigger points in the upper trapezius muscle and reduces pain in subjects with chronic myofascial pain. *PM&R*, *7*(7), pp. 711–718.

Goodwin, J.E., Glaister, M., Howatson, G., Lockey, R.A. and McInnes, G., 2007. Effect of preperformance lower-limb massage on thirty-meter sprint running. *Journal of Strength and Conditioning Research*, *21*(4), p. 1028.

Govus, A.D., Andersson, E.P., Shannon, O.M., Provis, H., Karlsson, M. and McGawley, K., 2018. Commercially available compression garments or electrical stimulation do not enhance recovery following a sprint competition in elite cross-country skiers. *European Journal of Sport Science*, *18*(10), pp. 1299–1308.

Jay, K., Sundstrup, E., Søndergaard, S.D., Behm, D., Brandt, M., Særvoll, C.A., Jakobsen, M.D. and Andersen, L.L., 2014. Specific and cross over effects of massage for muscle soreness: Randomized controlled trial. *International Journal of Sports Physical Therapy*, 9(1):82–91.

Jooste, K., Khumalo, V. and Maritz, J., 2013. Sportmen's experiences at a somatology clinic receiving a sport massage. *Health SA Gesondheid (Online)*, *18*(1), pp. 1–9.

Kidd, R.F. 2009. Why myofascial release will never be evidence-based. *International Musculoskeletal Medicine*, *31*(2), pp. 55–56.

Kim, J., Sung, D.J. and Lee, J., 2017. Therapeutic effectiveness of instrument-assisted soft tissue mobilization for soft tissue injury: Mechanisms and practical application. *Journal of Exercise Rehabilitation*, *13*(1), p. 12.

Kim, J.I., Lee, M.S., Lee, D.H., Boddy, K. and Ernst, E., 2011. Cupping for treating pain: A systematic review. *Evidence-Based Complementary and Alternative Medicine*, *2011*. Article ID 467014. doi:10.1093/ecam/nep035

Krueger, M., Costello, J.T., Achtzehn, S., Dittmar, K.H. and Mester, J., 2019. Whole-body cryotherapy (−110 C) following high-intensity intermittent exercise does not alter hormonal, inflammatory or muscle damage biomarkers in trained males. *Cytokine*, *113*, pp. 277–284.

Lee, D.C., Sheridan, S., Ali, A., Sutanto, D. and Wong, S.H., 2021. Wearing compression tights post-exercise enhances recovery hemodynamics and subsequent cycling performance. *European Journal of Applied Physiology*, *121*(7), pp. 2091–2100.

McKechnie, G.J., Young, W.B. and Behm, D.G., 2007. Acute effects of two massage techniques on ankle joint flexibility and power of the plantar flexors. *Journal of Sports Science & Medicine*, *6*(4), p. 498.

Nunes, G.S., Bender, P.U., de Menezes, F.S., Yamashitafuji, I., Vargas, V.Z. and Wageck, B., 2016. Massage therapy decreases pain and perceived fatigue after long-distance Ironman triathlon: A randomised trial. *Journal of Physiotherapy*, *62*(2), pp. 83–87.

Pearcey, G.E., Bradbury-Squires, D.J., Kawamoto, J.E., Drinkwater, E.J., Behm, D.G. and Button, D.C., 2015. Foam rolling for delayed-onset muscle soreness and recovery of dynamic performance measures. *Journal of Athletic Training*, *50*(1), pp. 5–13.

Romero-Moraleda, B., La Touche, R., Lerma-Lara, S., Ferrer-Peña, R., Paredes, V., Peinado, A.B. and Muñoz-García, D., 2017. Neurodynamic mobilization and foam rolling improved delayed-onset muscle soreness in a healthy adult population: A randomized controlled clinical trial. *PeerJ*, *5*, p. e3908.

Rose, C., Edwards, K.M., Siegler, J., Graham, K. and Caillaud, C., 2017. Whole-body cryotherapy as a recovery technique after exercise: A review of the literature. *International Journal of Sports Medicine*, *38*(14), pp. 1049–1060.

Sarli, D. and Agus, M., 2014. Research articles the effect of differences oxytocin levels through oxytocin massage against number of bleeding in mother 2 hours postpartum. *Jurnal Kesehatan Andalas*, *4*(3), pp. 743–750.

Szabo, A., Rendi, M., Szabó, T., Velenczei, A. and Kovács, Á., 2008. Psychological effects of massage on running. *Journal of Social, Behavioral, and Health Sciences*, *2*(1), p. 1.

Visconti, L., Capra, G., Carta, G., Forni, C. and Janin, D., 2015. Effect of massage on DOMS in ultramarathon runners: A pilot study. *Journal of Bodywork and Movement Therapies*, *19*(3), pp. 458–463.

Wilson, L.J., Dimitriou, L., Hills, F.A., Gondek, M.B. and Cockburn, E., 2019. Whole body cryotherapy, cold water immersion, or a placebo following resistance exercise: A case of mind over matter? *European Journal of Applied Physiology*, *119*(1), pp. 135–147.

Zusman, M., 2013. Belief reinforcement: one reason why costs for low back pain have not decreased. *Journal of Multidisciplinary Healthcare*, *6*, pp. 197.

Index